The Premed Playbook
Guide to the Medical School Interview

ENDORSEMENTS

"Dr. Gray has compiled a very detailed, comprehensive, and practical book on the medical school interview. What makes this book so unique is his emphasis on the introspective process. Instead of simply providing a checklist of do's and don'ts, he challenges the reader to examine their strengths and weaknesses and gives them a blueprint on how to put their best foot forward. His advice is real-world and compiled by many interviewers, including myself, who have years of experience interviewing medical school applicants. I highly recommend this book as a fundamental preparation tool for the application process."

Gregory M. Polites, MD
Associate Professor of Emergency Medicine
Chairman of the Central Subcommittee on Admissions
Washington University School of Medicine

"*The Premed Playbook* is a must-have for every future doctor's collection. Great advice, comprehensive, and to the point. Dr. Gray breaks it down, play by play.

Sujay Kansagra, MD
Author of *The Medical School Manual,*
Everything I Learned in Medical School,
and *Why Medicine*"

"Dr. Gray offers a simple and concise guide to having a successful medical school interview. Having been through the medical school process three times while applying and then serving on the admissions committee during my last year of medical school, I know what it takes to have a successful interview. I highly recommend this book for every student to read and have available for reference during the medical school interview season."

Antonio J. Webb, MD
Author of *Overcoming the Odds*

THE PREMED PLAYBOOK

GUIDE TO THE MEDICAL SCHOOL INTERVIEW

Be Prepared, Perform Well, Get Accepted

Ryan Gray, MD

NEW YORK

NASHVILLE • MELBOURNE • VANCOUVER

The Premed Playbook Guide to the
Medical School Interview

Be Prepared, Perform Well, Get Accepted

Published in New York, New York, by Morgan James Publishing. Morgan James is a trademark of Morgan James, LLC. www.MorganJamesPublishing.com

The Morgan James Speakers Group can bring authors to your live event. For more information or to book an event visit The Morgan James Speakers Group at www.TheMorganJamesSpeakersGroup.com.

ISBN 9781683502159 paperback
ISBN 9781683502166 eBook
ISBN 9781683502173 hardcover
Library of Congress Control Number: 2016914310

Cover Design by:
Rachel Lopez
www.r2cdesign.com

Interior Design by:
Chris Treccani
www.3dogdesign.net

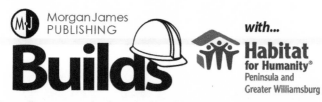

In an effort to support local communities, raise awareness and funds, Morgan James Publishing donates a percentage of all book sales for the life of each book to Habitat for Humanity Peninsula and Greater Williamsburg.

Get involved today! Visit
www.MorganJamesBuilds.com

To my amazing wife, Allison,
for supporting me on this journey.

DOWNLOAD 3 FULL MOCK INTERVIEWS FOR FREE

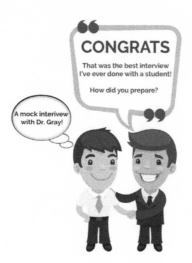

READ THIS FIRST

Just to say thanks for purchasing my book, I would like to give you 3 full mock interview recordings, 100% FREE!

CLICK HERE TO DOWNLOAD

(or go to: http://www.medschoolinterviewbook.com/freedownload)

DISCLOSURE

Some links in this book are affiliate links. If you end up using the product I recommend (I only recommend products I trust), I get some beer money.

TABLE OF CONTENTS

Introduction   *xiii*

Section I	**The Knowledge**	**xvii**
Chapter 1	The Process Leading up to the Interview	1
Chapter 2	Why It's Important	5
Chapter 3	Why You Didn't Get an Interview	7
Chapter 4	Different is Better Than Better	11
Chapter 5	Core Competencies and Holistic Review	15
Chapter 6	Types of Interviews	21
Chapter 7	Before the Interview	27
Chapter 8	After the Interview	35
Chapter 9	Common Mistakes	39
Chapter 10	How to Succeed	47
Chapter 11	Mock Interview Prep	49
Section II	**The Questions**	**53**
Chapter 12	Opening Questions	55

Chapter 13   Grades and MCAT Score Questions   57
Chapter 14   Extracurricular Activities Questions   59
Chapter 15   "Why Medicine?" Questions   61
Chapter 16   Ethical and Moral Questions   63
Chapter 17   Politics, Policy and Healthcare Questions   69
Chapter 18   'Your Future' Questions   75
Chapter 19   Personal Questions   77
Chapter 20   School Related Questions   83
Chapter 21   Miscellaneous Questions   85
Chapter 22   Multiple Mini Interview Scenarios   93
Chapter 23   Questions to Ask the Interviewer   99
Chapter 24   Questions to Ask the Medical Students   101

Section III   The Examples   105
Chapter 25   Tell Me About Yourself   107
Chapter 26   Any Red Flags?   127
Chapter 27   Why Medicine?   135
Chapter 28   Why Not Nurse or PA?   147
Chapter 29   Why DO?   151
Chapter 30   What is Your Biggest Weakness?   157
Chapter 31   What is the Biggest Challenge Facing Healthcare?   163
Chapter 32   What do you Think About the ACA?   167
Chapter 33   Talk About Your Poor Grades   173
Chapter 34   What are your Thoughts on Abortion? (And Other Ethical
              and Moral Questions)   177
Chapter 35   Why Should We Pick You?   185

Closing   199
About the Author   203
Resources   205
References   209

INTRODUCTION

Little did I know, when I was interviewing for medical school many years ago, that I would now be teaching other students how to successfully prepare for their own medical school interviews.

Like some of you, I went to a large state school—the University of Florida. Even though the majority of premed advisors are working hard to give you the best guidance available, I was just another number on my advisor's roster. This led to her not knowing me very well, if at all. I was told by my advisor not to apply to medical school. Her advice was not based on my GPA (I finished with a 3.73 science GPA), and it was not based on my Medical College Admissions Test (MCAT) (I hadn't taken it yet). I was told not to apply to medical school because I was a white male. She said that there were too many of 'us' applying.

Hopefully, your school (assuming you are in school) has a great premed advising office. While my experience was definitely rough, these advisors are working hard to make sure that they are making you as successful as possible. Please use them as your first stop in gathering information. They know you, your school, and are there to give you feedback specific to you.

Needless to say, I didn't seek out much more advice from her and was left to navigate the last two years of my undergraduate studies on my own. Luckily, I was surrounded by a group of amazing friends and classmates who were also premed, and we collectively sought out as much information as we could find that could help us prepare for medical school.

The first time I applied to medical school, it was the first year the American Medical College Application Service (AMCAS) process was online. All the students applying that year were unluckily blessed with using software that probably wasn't ready for release. It took multiple attempts to enter in information, only to be left with a blank screen and nothing saved at the end. Finally, after the grueling process, I submitted my application, only to learn that the computer system transmitting the application to the schools had its own glitches.

The Association of American Medical Colleges (AAMC) had to print out all of the applications and mail them to each of the schools that had been applied to. Unfortunately, this was during the anthrax scare in 2001, which shut down the mail service in D.C.—where the AAMC is located. Even after all of that, I was still a strong enough applicant to have received two interviews, one at the University of Florida where I was an undergrad, and the other at the University of Colorado.

I remember how nervous I was on each of the interview days. I remember going in thinking that I didn't belong there, that there must have been a mistake; the staff was going to find out when I checked in that I really didn't have an interview. It wasn't a mistake. I had my interviews, and the days went as smoothly as I could have hoped for. I remember walking around the campus during the tour in awe of my surroundings, giddy that one day I was going to be a student here, just like all of the medical students I saw roaming the halls. I thought the interviews went well, but I guess they weren't good enough. I wasn't accepted at either school. I didn't even make a waitlist. I was crushed and didn't think I was going to be able to become a physician.

After doing some research, I found out that, to be a more competitive applicant, there were some items lacking in my application. For starters, I needed formal shadowing experience, which I hadn't had before. I mostly had done traditional volunteer work at the hospital—working at the information desk showing people where the elevators were, and transporting patients to and from different tests and procedures.

Shadowing, as I know now, is a valuable tool to help you gain insight into what life is like as a physician. It's not clinical or hands-on experience, but it allows you to get close to the action, and see what your life may look like in the future. Admissions committees want to make sure you know what you are getting yourself into (and aren't basing the next 7+ years of your life on scenes from Grey's Anatomy).

Two years later, after moving to Colorado and finding an orthopedic surgeon to shadow (ok, my mom found him), I reapplied to medical school. This time the computer systems were working well, but I only received one interview invite. It was from New York Medical College (NYMC). The interview day went well. I had a higher sense of appreciation this time around, because of the past rejections. It meant a lot more to me this time. I wanted it more. I needed it more. And this time, they wanted me too.

At the time of my acceptance, I was working as a Fitness Program Manager for a gym in Boston. That job gave me amazing experience managing other people and running a business—two skills I thought would be valuable one day as a physician. I contacted NYMC and asked that I be allowed to defer one year and enter with the class of 2009 instead of 2008. They agreed. That decision had a significant impact on my life because it was during orientation week in 2005 that I met Allison, who is now my wife. I went on to complete my four years at NYMC on an Air Force scholarship, I did a one-year transitional internship in the Boston area, and completed five years of active duty military service with the United States Air Force.

In 2012, knowing that there was a severe lack of good information about the premed process online, I started the Medical School Headquarters to help premed students, like you, navigate the path to medical school. I want you to have the expert advice that I didn't have. I want to provide you with advice that I have gathered from the experts, from those who are actually making admissions decisions, and not just other premeds. The Premed Years podcast has given me the opportunity to interview former and current deans of medical schools and other Admissions Committee members. I want you to see that getting into medical school is possible, even if you've made mistakes along the way.

This book focuses on the medical school interview process: I'm going to help you understand the importance of the interview, teach you strategies to prepare for it, make sure you make the most of the day, and teach you the different categories of questions, as well as some frameworks on how to answer each category. I do want you to understand one thing though—it doesn't matter how many books you read about the medical school interview, if you don't put in the effort to practice, then you're setting yourself up for disaster. Don't worry though—we'll cover ways for you to get the practice you need. If you read this book and dedicate the time to practice, then an acceptance to medical school is closer than you can imagine. I can't guarantee that you will be accepted into medical school just from reading this book, but I can guarantee that you will be better prepared for interview day.

SECTION I

THE KNOWLEDGE

CHAPTER 1

THE PROCESS LEADING UP TO THE INTERVIEW

I'm not going to cover the entire premed process in this book, but I do want to provide you with some basic insight so you know what to expect with the application process leading up to your interview. Texas has their own medical school application service, the Texas Medical & Dental School Application Service (TMDSAS), and their timeline is slightly different but close enough that I won't address it separately. The other two application services, the American Medical College Application (AMCAS), and the American Association of Colleges of Osteopathic Medicine Application Service (AACOMAS) are the application services for MD schools and DO schools, respectively.

The application process opens up in May the year before you plan on starting medical school. You are given approximately a month to fill in the information needed to apply, which includes grades, extracurricular activities, demographics, your personal statement and other miscellaneous information. At the beginning of June, you can submit your primary applications for verification. Your transcripts, which you need to have submitted to each of the application services, are compared to the grades that you manually entered. After your application is verified and the application service has done their part, they will submit your application to each of the schools you selected. This process typically takes place starting the last week of June, assuming you submitted your application early—which you should plan on.

After you submit your primary applications, most of the medical schools you apply to will send you a secondary application to fill out. Depending on the school's policies, some will do this even without looking at your initial application. Secondary applications usually consist of more essays. Some examples of these include describing any gaps in your education, describing your desire to attend that medical school, your understanding and experience with diversity and describing a challenging situation that you've had to overcome. You'll want to turn these essays in as soon as possible. Secondary applications are expensive; you can expect to pay about $100 for each secondary application.

After your secondary applications have been submitted, your work is done—assuming your MCAT scores have been released. If you are still waiting on an MCAT test date or a score to be released, some schools will wait for your score before they review your application. Once your application is complete, the school will review it and will decide whether or not you will be invited for an interview. These invitations will be sent via email, so make sure you are using a valid email address when you submit your application.

Most medical schools use what is known as a rolling admissions process, which I like to compare to a big game of musical chairs. Due to the fact that each school offers a limited number of interviews, the longer you wait to submit your application, and the later your MCAT scores are released, the less likely you are to obtain an invitation for an interview. If they are reviewing your application later in the cycle, they have already invited many students and are getting close to filling all of their interview slots.

The day you receive your first interview invite is a great day. It's a day you've worked so hard to get to. You've sacrificed a lot to get the interview, but the work isn't over yet. Let's talk about why the medical school interview is so important and how to best prepare for it.

CHAPTER 2

WHY IT'S IMPORTANT

The medical school interview gives the Admissions Committee an opportunity to learn more about you as a person, and not just what is in your application. It gives them the ability to judge how well you may fit into the rest of the entering class. It allows them to listen to you, observe you, and communicate with you.

With thousands of applications coming into each medical school every year, there has to be a way for the school to figure out who they are going to accept and who they are going to reject. Much of this initial process is done automatically based on filters that schools can set with the application software. Some schools claim that they review *every* application, but what they don't tell you is that they are likely sorting the applications based on GPA and MCAT, and if your scores are below average, there's a good chance that the Admissions Committee will never review your application. But, if you do get that golden ticket, and receive an interview invite, the school has determined that you are a candidate worthy of further consideration.

Reviewing information available on a few medical school websites, the percentage of applicants at each school who are invited for an interview is low, only about 15-20%. For example, according to Albert Einstein College of Medicine's 2015-2016 Applicant Guide[1], they interviewed about 16% of their applicants (1,324 students out of 8,138 applications). If you received an interview invite, then you are way ahead of the game.

Here's why the interview is so important. You have to assume the mindset that the acceptance is yours to lose when you receive an interview invite. While that may be stretching the truth a little, the fact is that the school thinks your grades are good enough. Your extracurricular activities are good enough. Your letters of recommendation are good enough. What else is there? All that is left is *you*! Can you still get in if you bomb your interview, even with an amazing application? Probably not. If you don't shine, but don't fail the interview, will you still have a chance if the rest of your application is great? There's a good chance. Medical schools understand the amount of stress you are under. They understand that the interview process can be subjective. They try their best to remove those variables, but people are still people, and the person interviewing you has his or her own biases. Most interviews consist of you meeting with multiple interviewers, so if you don't do well with one, you will need to mentally reset and go into the next interview fresh and confident. The best golfers in the world are the ones who can make a bad shot and forget about it as soon they are ready for the next shot. You need to have this mindset too.

At the end of the day, you need to go in prepared to be yourself and be confident. Make the committee members have no choice but to believe in you. Leave them no choice but to believe in you.

CHAPTER 3

WHY YOU DIDN'T GET AN INTERVIEW

If you didn't get an interview from a school that you assumed you would, then you made a very common mistake. There is no such thing as a safety school or fallback school. Here are some things to keep in mind. Medical schools are always looking for students who they believe will be academically successful. If your grades or MCAT scores don't show them that you can be successful as a student, you won't get an interview. If you are applying to a large number of public schools as an out-of-state applicant, you are fighting an uphill battle. State schools almost always look to admit state residents. Some schools are looking for students interested in primary care. Some are seeking students who want to practice in rural areas. What exactly they are looking for, nobody knows except for them.

In addition to the unknown factors that each school is looking for, you're also dealing with individual biases from each member of the Admissions Committee.

Each person has their own experiences and set of lenses that they are looking through as they review your application. It could be the B- you got in organic chemistry, or that substandard MCAT score, or perhaps you are missing that one truly outstanding extracurricular activity that they were looking for. This is why it's so important to apply broadly to many different schools and not just the ones that you think you have a shot at. I've seen great applications from students who should have received an acceptance, but who only applied to one school, thereby severely limiting their chances of being accepted.

The most common reason for not getting accepted to medical school, according to some Admissions Committee members, is a lack of enough clinical exposure. Remember, schools need to make sure you understand what you are getting yourself into. Medical school and being a physician isn't what it seems to be from watching an episode of Grey's Anatomy or Scrubs. Unlike shadowing, which is what I was missing in my application, clinical experience puts you up front and center with the patient. Just because you like science and want to help people doesn't mean you will actually like helping sick people. Clinical experience will help you figure that out and give confidence to the Admissions Committee that you are in fact ready for this career.

Of course, there are some major red flags that, if present in your application, might cause a school to not invite you for an interview. These red flags can include: criminal records including DUI or other arrests, or disciplinary actions from your university due to plagiarism or other infractions. These are questions on the application that you have to answer, so it's very easy for the school to put your application into the "Do Not Interview" pile, just for marking 'Yes' in one of those boxes. Of course, I've also seen students with red flags in their application receive an interview invitation and gain their acceptance. Kain was one student I interviewed on The Premed Years podcast. He was academically dismissed from his undergrad program his first time through. Many years later, he wanted to go back and give medical school another shot. He had to work hard and jump through some hoops, but after all of that hard work, he earned an acceptance to the University of Central Florida College of Medicine. You can hear his story at http://medicalschoolhq.net/174.

If your GPA and MCAT scores are drastically below the school's average, it is unlikely that you will get an interview. Use the Medical School Admission Requirements[2] (MSAR) service from the AAMC and the College Information Book[3] (CIB) from the AACOM to see what the averages are for the schools you are interested in applying to.

There is a general rule of thumb that circulates online which compares your MCAT and GPA scores to a specific school, determining whether or not you should apply. I, however, don't believe in this rule of thumb. You have a 0% chance of getting into a school that you don't apply to, and a higher chance of getting in if you do apply. There may be something in your application which will entice an admissions committee member to overlook a poor MCAT score or a low GPA. The average number of schools that students apply to according to both the AAMC and AACOM is about 15[4] and 9[5], respectively. This means that students who are applying to both MD and DO schools are applying to an average of 24 schools. The total number of schools that you apply to should be determined by where you are interested in going, your strength as an applicant, and your budget. The cost of applying to medical school adds up very quickly. Don't be surprised if it ends up costing you several thousand dollars to apply and travel for your interviews. This is another good reason why you need to prepare yourself in the best way possible.

If you don't get an interview, you can always try to advocate for yourself by reaching out to the school and requesting them to reconsider their initial decision. You will need to effectively convince the school that you are a worthy candidate, and why they should look past any sort of red flags that may be putting your application in the wrong pile.

I coached one student to help him prepare for an interview at Wake Forest. He didn't get an interview initially because he was rejected before that stage. But when his fiancée was accepted, he immediately wrote a letter and overnighted it to the dean of admissions. He had an interview invite that same week, and an acceptance letter soon after his interview. The school didn't accept him because of his fiancée, but they did give his application a second chance because of it.

Some schools will offer an application review in which they will talk to you and let you know why you didn't get an interview. Not every school offers this, and sometimes the review will have to be delayed due to the application cycle and volume of applicants, but you can request it.

When you don't receive an invitation for an interview, there is most likely something in your application that medical schools don't like. You need to figure out what it is, fix it, and reapply. Being a reapplicant is not a bad thing; it won't hurt your chances of getting into medical school—with one caveat: There are some medical schools that will restrict you from applying more than two or three times. You really need to do your research into each school to know each of their requirements and restrictions. The best place to do this is on each school's website.

I did a great interview with a former dean of admissions about being a reapplicant. You can find that interview at http://medicalschoolhq.net/171.

CHAPTER 4

DIFFERENT IS BETTER THAN BETTER

What truly separates each applicant? What separates those who get into medical school from those who are left holding rejection letters? I wish it were as simple as giving you a checklist and telling you that if you check every box, you will have an acceptance to medical school. Unfortunately, it's not that easy. As discussed in the previous chapter, every school is looking for specific attributes in the students who will make up their next class. If you don't possess those attributes, then you might not be accepted, regardless of your MCAT and GPA scores. It's often said that you need to stand out in your application to get in. But what does that really mean? Does it mean you need a 4.0 GPA, a 528 on the MCAT, and thousands of hours of shadowing and volunteer experience?

Schools are not looking for the perfect applicant. They are looking for a student who has demonstrated that he or she is able to handle the medical school curriculum, do well in residency, and more importantly, be a good human being who is willing to put others before him or herself. These are the attributes that make up a great applicant to medical school, and ultimately a great physician.

Nontraditional students have an advantage when it comes to demonstrating many of the traits that medical schools are looking for. Traditional students have been locked up in school for all of their lives without gaining much real-world experience. Nontraditional students, on the other hand, have been out in the workforce, may have traveled the world, and have first-hand knowledge of what it's like to not be a student. This allows the nontraditional students to more easily build rapport with patients.

What can separate you, regardless of whether you're a traditional or nontraditional student, is YOU. If every applicant to medical school has a 3.5 GPA and 520 on the MCAT, how will the schools choose who gets in and who does not? Each person, the person behind the numbers, is what separates every application—your experiences, childhood, good times, bad times, personality, and communication skills. Each of your individual traits is what separates you from your fellow classmates. Don't make excuses that you lead a boring life. It's *your* life; it is what makes you different. Yes, if you don't put in any effort and you go to class and go home, you're not going to set yourself apart. You need to explore the world with your own eyes, not go through life checking off boxes assuming that doing just that will get you into medical school. You need to create opportunities that will allow you to expand your horizons and increase your life experiences, all while trying to juggle school, friendships, family and more.

How can you start to do that? Well, if you're a nontraditional student, you've already done that. The mere fact that you're a nontraditional student has made you different. Jessica, for example, was a nontraditional premed student. Having already gone to college to pursue acting, she was living in Los Angeles, working as an actress when health problems struck her dad. Through her interactions with his physicians, her desires changed. She went back to college and completed her medical school prerequisites through a post-baccalaureate program. She applied broadly to medical schools and went on 11 interviews. She received ten acceptances and was waitlisted at the 11th (I wonder what that 11th school was thinking!). You can hear more about her story at http://medicalschoolhq. net/168. Yes, her grades and her MCAT score were good. But good grades and a good MCAT score don't earn you ten acceptances. Her story and her experiences earned her that. She earned ten acceptances by knowing what made her different and by highlighting that on her application and during her interviews. Together, we worked hard crafting her personal statement and honing her interview responses during her mock interview prep. When I followed up with her, she talked about her interviews and how the interviewers wanted to talk about her acting career and not her academics. Acting was something different, and that's what they were drawn to.

If you're a traditional student, look at what Alex did at the University of Florida with his Dream Team project (http://medicalschoolhq.net/83). Alex, an undergraduate student, co-founded the Dream Team after seeing a need at a local hospital. He did the work, and now several years later his creation has contributed over 5,000 hours of direct volunteering time to help support the kids in the hospital. Alex is different.

Joshua Dawson, Yarid Mera, and Jawwad Ali are other traditional students making names for themselves by being different. They have worked to set up a system to help other premed students find physicians to shadow[6]. They are different. And so are you!

CHAPTER 5

CORE COMPETENCIES AND HOLISTIC REVIEW

The AAMC has a list of 15 core competencies[7] for entering medical students, which medical schools use to help them determine which students to accept. These core competencies are broken down into four categories: interpersonal, intrapersonal, thinking and reasoning, and science. While these core competencies have been developed to help guide admissions to medical school, don't use this as an exhaustive list of what you need to have in order to be accepted. Some schools may be looking for more than these 15 competencies, while some schools may be looking at fewer.

These competencies are provided not as a checklist to make sure that you meet each of them, but so you can understand how medical schools may be evaluating you during your interview day, and even before that as they evaluate your application.

Interpersonal Competencies

Service orientation, social skills, cultural competence, teamwork and oral communication are all included in the interpersonal competencies.

Service Orientation: This competency is demonstrated by showing a desire to help others and your ability to respond to other people's needs, feelings and emotions. It shows that you understand how you fit into society on a larger scale, and how your actions affect those around you. This is demonstrated through your extracurricular activities. What have you done that shows you are willing to put others before yourself? Who have you positively affected with your volunteering? What impact did you make on the people you were serving?

Question that may be asked: "Tell me about your most impactful volunteering experience."

Social Skills: This is a competency that outside of an interview is hard to judge. Your letter writers will hopefully speak to this, but ultimately your interview is how this competency is judged. The interviewers, as well as all the staff, at the medical school are watching your interactions with others, watching how aware you are of other people and what their needs and feelings are. How do you respond to their cues, and do you treat everyone with respect?

Cultural Competence: Every day the U.S. becomes more and more diverse. As a physician, you will be treating people from all walks of life and will need to demonstrate an understanding of socio-cultural factors that affect you and your patients. You need to show respect and appreciation for the differences in people. Pay close attention to this one because there was a study published in 2016 that showed Caucasian medical students have very wrong beliefs about the biological differences between Caucasians and African Americans.

Question that may be asked: "Tell me about a time you had to alter what you were doing to meet a diversity need or challenge?"

Teamwork: The healthcare team involves many different people all working together to provide each patient with the best care possible; these include: physicians from multiple specialties, nurses, social workers, physical therapists, to name a few. You need to demonstrate the ability to work collaboratively with others to achieve the best possible outcomes for each patient.

Question that may be asked: "Tell me about a time you worked collaboratively with a team to accomplish something."

Oral Communication: Like Social Skills, this competency is hard to judge outside of an interview. Communicating with patients, their families, and other healthcare team members is essential for the best possible patient care.

Intrapersonal Competencies

Ethical responsibility to self and others, reliability and dependability, resilience and adaptability, and capacity for improvement are included in the intrapersonal competencies.

Ethical Responsibility to Self and Others: If you've had any sort of run-in with the police or academic issues at your school, you will have trouble proving to the Admissions Committee that you are ethically responsible. Your integrity is not only important for medicine—it's important as a human being.

Question that may be asked: "Tell me about a time you did something bad and got in trouble for it."

Reliability and Dependability: Being reliable to your patients and the other members of the healthcare team is vital for the best possible patient care. If people can't trust that you will do what you say, or will be somewhere when you say you'll be there, they will have a hard time relying on you.

Question that may be asked: "Tell me about a time you weren't as dependable as you wanted to be."

Resilience and Adaptability: If you've ever experienced a poor semester and bounced back, or had family situations cause stress at home that impacted your ability to perform well in school, you'll be able to discuss this easily. The truth is we all have to adapt every day. Life doesn't always go as planned. If you're at the interview stage, then you have probably handled this well. Now it's just time to discuss it during the interview.

Question that may be asked: "Tell me about a time you needed to adapt to a situation to accomplish a goal."

Capacity for Improvement: If you've been out of school for a little while, what did you do with your time? Did you do anything that challenged you intellectually, or did you play video games every day? Did you seek out opportunities for continued learning while in school? Did you learn new hobbies or skills? Have you read a book recently?

Question that may be asked: "Tell me about the most recent book you've read."

Thinking and Reasoning Competencies

Critical thinking, quantitative reasoning, scientific inquiry, and written communication are included in the thinking and reasoning competencies.

Critical Thinking: This one is pretty straightforward. As a physician, you'll be required to use a great deal of logic and reasoning to determine solutions to problems.

Question that may be asked: "Tell me about a time you had to come up with a unique solution to a problem."

Quantitative Reasoning: This is another one that is pretty straightforward. The ability to use math and apply it to explain the world around you shows a certain level of intelligence.

Scientific Inquiry: The scientific process is core to being a physician, and to the research necessary in the medical field. You should be able to integrate information and synthesize new knowledge to solve problems, formulate, and test research questions and hypotheses.

Question that may be asked: "Tell me what you were testing with the research experiment you were involved in."

Written Communication: How well you can communicate both orally and through written word is a key marker of your ability to effectively work as a physician.

Science Competencies

Living systems and human behavior are a part of the science competencies.

Living Systems: You should be able to apply your knowledge and skills learned in school to solve problems around livings systems like organs, cells, and molecules. This competency is more reflected in your grades and MCAT score.

Human Behavior: Using your knowledge of our social systems to help solve problems around psychology, socio-cultural and biological factors that affect our health and well-being is just as important as the ability to apply the living systems knowledge. This is a new emphasis on the MCAT and in medical school, and it is also more reflected in your grades and MCAT score.

Holistic Review

Several years ago, the AAMC[8] set out to give medical schools tools they could use to help assess applicants, understanding that each student brings his or her own strengths and weaknesses based on the diversity of their upbringing. It helps schools balance factors like experiences, personal attributes, and academic performances. It also helps standardize some aspects of the admissions process which is a good thing for everyone.

Using a holistic review allows the diversity of the medical school class to hopefully better reflect the diversity of society as a whole. It is beneficial to all involved to have physicians aware of the unique aspects of the many different cultures we have represented in the United States.

CHAPTER 6

TYPES OF INTERVIEWS

There are several types of interviews that you may be asked to participate in. Each school selects the type of interview that will best utilize their resources, and help them in choosing the best students to make up their next class. You will know, from your research, or just by asking, what type of interview you are walking into. There shouldn't be any surprises here.

Each type of interview focuses on different questions, different preparation and different skills necessary to do your best. Ultimately, doing well on your interview day comes down to good communication skills and answering the questions in a calm, confident way, which is something that you can learn with practice during your mock interviews.

Later on in the book, there will be specific questions as well as Multiple Mini Interview (MMI) scenarios which you can use to help you prepare for your interview.

Let's talk about the different types of interviews.

Open-file Interview

The open-file, or open interview, is an interview in which the interviewer has access to your complete application. This does not necessarily mean that they have read your entire application, or that they know everything that is in your application. You may be asked to answer questions that you think are a waste of time because if the interviewer would just look at your application, he or she would know the answer. If you are asked a question like this, you should answer the questions as if the interviewer doesn't know what's in your application. Remember, just because they have access to it, doesn't mean they have read it. I've talked to interviewers who, even though it's an open interview, prefer to go into the interview as if it were blind.

Be prepared to talk in depth about your personal statement, your secondary application essays, every one of your grades, every one of your extracurricular activities, and your MCAT score. The interviewer can ask you a question about anything that he or she sees in your application. It is imperative that you know your application inside and out. You should know why you entered certain extracurricular activities and why you included what you wrote in your personal statement. Nothing looks worse than being asked about one of your extracurricular activities and not being prepared to talk about it.

Closed-file or Partial-file Interview

Also known as the blind interview, the closed-file interview is one in which the interviewer has no access to your application. He or she does not know your GPA, your MCAT score, or anything else about you.

In the partial-file interview, the interviewer knows certain parts of your application, typically your personal statement, extracurricular activities and secondary essay responses.

In these types of interviews, the interviewer may be more conversational because he or she is just looking to connect with you instead of picking apart your application. You may be asked generic questions like 'tell me about yourself,' or 'tell me about any red flags I may find in your application when I go and review it later.'

The closed-file or partial-file interviews allow you to steer the conversation a bit more because the interviewer isn't being distracted with questions she thinks she has to ask based on your application. Knowing how to tell your story is imperative with this style of interview. Working hard during your mock interviews will allow you to tell your story in such a way that the interviewer will ask more questions based on what you just said. For example, if you bring up that you were a collegiate tennis player and won a championship, and the interviewer is a tennis fan, you've just allowed for the interview to go into a discussion about tennis. This type of interaction allows the interviewer to connect with you on a personal level, and not just as another applicant to medical school.

The more you can bring *you* into the discussion, the better off you are. Don't recite your extracurricular list. Don't give a timeline of your life. Going through this question over multiple sessions of mock interviews will bring out your best answers! In Section III, you'll see answers from students over the course of several mock interview sessions with me, and how they changed and improved with my feedback.

Panel Interview

In the panel interview, it can seem like the world is crashing down on you. In this interview, there are several interviewers who have the ability to ask you questions. These interviewers can be from various parts of the faculty of the medical school, or from the hospital affiliated with the school. There can even be a medical student who is part of the panel. You should treat this interview no differently than any of the other interviews. Listen carefully when being asked questions; maintain good eye contact with the person asking you a question; make sure that when you are talking, you make eye contact with all of the panel members.

Group Interview

Similar to the panel interview, group interviews will typically have several interviewers, but this time instead of just you answering the questions, there will be several other students being interviewed as well.

The goal here is to show respect for the other students who are being interviewed. This is not your time to show your dominance. You need to listen carefully to the answers that are being given by other students and be prepared to follow up based on their answers. It is not a good time to zone out. Don't get stressed out if the panel asks each student the same question and the previous student has already given the answer you wanted to give. You can be lighthearted about it and mention that the answer was already given and try to expand as much as you can.

Multiple Mini Interview

The MMI is becoming more and more popular in the U.S. It was first created at McMaster University in Canada, and, at last count, there are approximately 50 schools in the U.S. using the Multiple Mini Interview. I had a good discussion with NYU's Dean Rivera about their transition to the MMI and how to best succeed during your MMI. You can listen to that podcast and see what he said at http://medicalschoolhq.net/152.

The MMI helps remove interviewer bias and has been shown to increase the quality of the students that a medical school ultimately accepts. Instead of having two people determine your fate, you have more opportunities to shine during your interview day. In addition, applicants with a more diverse background have more opportunities to allow that diversity to be demonstrated.

The MMI consists of many stations that assess your non-cognitive qualities, including empathy, communication skills, ethical decision making, critical thinking, knowledge of healthcare and current affairs, to name a few. Each school may have a different number of stations. I've seen numbers anywhere from seven to ten stations, but again, this isn't written in stone. Some schools may even work a traditional interview into the MMI day.

Prior to the start of the station, you are given a scenario to read over in a short period of time. You then enter the interview room and are greeted by the interviewer or actor in whatever role they are playing in that scenario. The actor could be the boss in the scenario, they could be the patient, or they could be a family member. The scenario will dictate how you respond and what the interviewer does according to those responses.

Each station interviewer usually has specific objectives by which they will judge you, and they will determine if those objectives are met. For instance, if you are talking to a nervous coworker, did you offer empathy, or did you go straight to trying to fix the situation without getting the proper input? Are you able to defend your ideas or discuss any issues that may have been raised? The interviewer or actor may challenge you to express your ideas as clearly as possible and defend your ideas in a stressful situation.

The good thing about the MMI is that if you do poorly in one station, you have several other stations to make up for that one bad one. If you don't connect with one interviewer, they are not going to derail your chance of getting into medical school if you are able to compose yourself and perform better the rest of the day.

Which One Is Best?

After you read all the details above, you may walk away with the question "Which type of interview is the best one?" or, "Which one is the easiest?" These are the wrong questions because you can't control what interview style the medical schools you are applying to will utilize. There are a lot of reasons to apply to a particular school, but the type of interview that they utilize should not be one of those reasons. The question you should be asking is how you can prepare for each of these interview styles because ultimately that is what is going to determine your success on interview day. Next, we'll dig into how to best prepare for your interview.

CHAPTER 7

BEFORE THE INTERVIEW

Congratulations! You have the golden ticket. The question now is what do you do to prepare? Soon after the excitement wears off, there is a lot of work that needs to be done to make sure that you can successfully prepare for your interview.

Researching the School

Research on your list of schools should be done before you apply, but if you have not already done this, now is the time to start researching each of the schools where you have an interview.

During the interview, you're going to be asked questions about why you want to go to that particular school. Generic answers like "it's a great school" or "the faculty here is amazing" are not good enough. Talking about how "the research opportunities excite me" doesn't say anything *specific* about the school. You could have said the exact same thing at any of your other interviews.

During mock interviews that I've done with students, I've heard everything from "I have family in the area," to the "reputation of the school is great." As the interviewer, if I can take your response and use it at any other medical school, your response is not specific enough to the school where you are interviewing. What you tell the interviewer should be so specific to that school that there is no possible way that you could be talking about any other medical school.

I helped two students, who were engaged at the time, prepare for their interviews at Wake Forest, and they had a very unique twist to this answer. They were both concert musicians turned premed students while studying for their doctoral degrees in music. Wake Forest has a medical professional's orchestra—the Triad Orchestra. They both easily said that one of the reasons that Wake Forest stood out to them was the orchestra and the opportunity to be involved in it. Now that is a very specific reason! They were also able to talk about other specific programs at the school. As a result, they both were accepted.

You should be able to talk about research that's happening at the school, specific programs that they offer, or even local and international relationships the school has that may provide you with opportunities to expand your work/experience beyond domestic and international borders.

I'm working with a student right now who lives in Utah, but she is originally from Ghana. She is very interested in the University of Utah School of Medicine, not only because that is where she lives, but because they have a very strong relationship with programs in Ghana. This will be an amazing opportunity for her to mention when she is asked why she is interested in attending the University of Utah.

Some other ideas include unique aspects of the curriculum or unique opportunities for patient interaction.

What Core Competencies Are They Looking for?

In the Core Competencies chapter, we listed each of the core competencies that the AAMC has published. Each school will typically adopt these and they may also add their own. As you are researching the school to prepare for your interview, see if you can find any published information on the school's specific criteria. You can also ask them directly.

Knowing the core competencies will help guide your thoughts when preparing your answers and your questions for interview day. The school will judge you based on how well you match into their core competency list. Being able to give them answers that make it easy for them to see that you fit will be a huge win for you.

Questions to Ask

You should have two sets of questions with you for each school you interview at—one set of questions are for the medical students, and the other set of questions are for the interviewers. The questions that you want to be prepared to ask the students involve things like activities, living situations, group dynamics, etc. If there are 3rd and 4th-year students around, you can ask questions about the rotations and hospitals. Asking the students about classes is also a good idea. Is attendance mandatory? What kind of note taking or lecture recording services are available? How often are tests administered?

The questions that you ask the interviewers are very important. Asking the right questions, to the right people, is key in finding the right answers. Many times students ask me the wrong questions during our mock interviews. They'll ask me questions about the curriculum, or questions about the student-run clinic. You have to understand that the interviewer may not have the answers to very specific questions like this.

Opinion-based questions, those that get the interviewer thinking and talking, are the best ones to ask here. Not only do you continue to have good dialogue, but hopefully you become a more memorable interviewee. One of my favorite questions is "If you had a daughter applying to medical school, would you hope they had this school as their number one choice, and why?" It's not something specific which the interviewer might not know about. It is a question that can give you some insight into how they view the school. Another favorite is, "If I were to poll the faculty about one opportunity they want the school to tackle, what would it be?" Notice how I used *opportunity* here instead of *challenge* or *obstacle*. Try to stay away from negative words on your interview day.

In Section II of the book, I'll provide more questions which you can ask interviewers during your interview day.

Looking the Part

You want to be memorable on the interview day, but not because of what you wear, the way you apply your makeup, or because of your hair style/color/etc.

Men

Men should wear a simple colored suit with a neutral shirt and a nice tie. You don't have to wear a black suit. If you don't own a suit, borrow one, rent one, or go buy one! If you have a fully grown out beard or mustache, you can keep it. If you have that 5 o'clock shadow look, shave it off. If it's the middle of #Movember and you're trying to support men's health, shave it off anyway! You can better support men's health with the skills you will have as a physician.

Women

The same (for the most part) applies to female applicants. Simple colors, skirt or pant suit, and nothing too low cut. Remember that there will probably be a lot of walking on the interview day so high heels probably aren't the most comfortable choice of shoe style.

Simple is the keyword for everything else—simple earrings that aren't too dangly and distracting, simple makeup with neutral colors, and simple hairstyles are what you want to stick to.

Getting There

In the military we had a saying, "early is on time, on time is late, and late is not acceptable." The last thing you want to do on your interview day is show up late. Plan on staying somewhere local the night before so you don't have to travel long distances in the morning. This will limit any chances of Murphy's Law kicking in, and allow you to get more rest the night before your interview. Schools will often have recommendations for accommodations available to you—you just need to ask.

Double and triple check the time that you need to be at the school. Double check the directions to the school. Find out from the school where you should park if you're driving, or where public transportation may drop you off. And, don't forget to check the weather! A simple black umbrella may save the day. If you can, take a drive by the school the day before your interview to get a lay of the land.

Plan on arriving at the school 30 minutes before the interview day starts. Walk around and enjoy the campus, talk to students or just hang out in your car. Find a mirror and give your clothes, makeup, and teeth one last check before heading to the office. You should arrive at the office 5-10 minutes before the scheduled start of the day.

What to Bring

The interview day is about you, the school, and the other interviewees. You shouldn't have any distractions with you or on you that may interrupt your day. Unless you are waiting for a call that your child is about to be born, or someone is about to pass, your phone should stay in the car or turned off in your briefcase or purse.

Remember how I said that you should expect that the acceptance is yours unless you do something to screw that up? Having your phone ring in the middle of the interview is one of those things that could impact your ability to be successful in the interview process.

Bring a bottle of water to stay hydrated, and maybe a small snack to keep your sugar levels up. A portfolio with some paper and a pen to take notes and write down contact information is a perfectly acceptable thing to bring with you to the interviews. You should have some of the questions that we talked about earlier written down on this too. Beyond these few things, there's not much more that you're going to need.

Know Your Application

This would seem like a no-brainer, but far too many students focus on others aspects of the interview and forget to review their application. You need to refresh your memory with what you said about yourself. Review each of your essays to remind yourself what you wrote about, not only in your personal statement but also in your secondary essay responses. Your list of extracurricular activities is another thing to review as well. Everything in your application is fair game. If you marked that you were fluent in Spanish, don't be caught off-guard if you are interviewed by a Spanish-speaking committee member who interviews you in Spanish.

Students can often get tripped up by the research experience they have participated in, so be prepared to answer questions explaining the research. You need to understand it and be prepared to explain it. An interviewer may ask you to explain your research in a way that a ten-year-old can understand it.

Knowing that interviewers can pick apart your application, you should always ask yourself this question before adding experiences into your application: Are you just adding the experience to fluff up your application and fill a spot, or were you very involved and can talk at length about the experience?

Ask for Input

As you begin your prep, it's best to start thinking about some of the most common questions that interviewers may ask about who you are. These questions can include your strengths, your weaknesses, and your unique qualities. Email your friends and family and ask them to answer these questions with you in mind. Tell them that you are preparing for your interviews and would like their insight. Doing this will allow you to see how other people perceive you. Let them know that you need the brutally honest truth and that no matter what they say, there will be no reprisal. Be careful with this exercise—sometimes you won't like the answers!

Read and Stay Connected

Knowing what is going on in the world is an important part of the interview. Remember, the committees want to make sure that you're a well-rounded person. This means knowing what is going on in the world. To accomplish this, reading is a must. Read about any current healthcare policy changes or news. Learn about Medicare, Medicaid, insurance costs, the future of medicine, physician debt, costs of medical care, etc.

There is an amazing app available for the iOS and Android operating systems called Texture[9]. This is a must have app to easily stay connected and informed about what is going on in the world. Texture lets you quickly search hundreds of magazines for one topic. For example, I did a search for "Affordable Care Act," and it came up with 589 magazine articles, all immediately available to read. Search for abortion, euthanasia, migrant crisis and more, and see what is being talked about. Texture helps you go beyond your comfort zone and gives you the ability to read different points of view that you would not normally read. This is very important on your interview journey (and in life in general). Check out the app by going to http://medicalschoolhq.net/texture.

CHAPTER 8

AFTER THE INTERVIEW

Time to put your feet up right? Not so fast! While the interview day may be over, you still have work to do.

During your interview day, you should be taking notes on the interactions that you've had with faculty and administration. With the notepad that you brought with you, make sure that you are writing down names throughout the day. You should also be taking notes about interesting discussions you had or topics you discussed, something that would be unique to you that you're hoping they'll remember later. Don't rely on your memory to recall who you interacted with and what you talked about. Your memory will fail you.

Thank You Notes

When you are back at a computer, it's time to start sending thank you notes to those that you had significant contact with on your interview day. You're not just thanking them for their time (remember many of the interviewers volunteer for the position); you're also helping them remember you. You should send thank you notes the same day that your interview took place. This shows that you are organized and prompt and that you care. Again, it is a way to help spark the mind of the interviewer and make them think about you again.

A good thank you note should be formal and include an appropriate greeting, a "thank you" early on in the note, something unique from your discussion, any last minute quality or trait that you want to highlight, and a solid close. In this age of Twitter and text messaging, you'd be surprised at how unprofessionally some students will communicate. While I talk about how the interview should be a coffee shop conversation between you and a future colleague, you want your note to convey respect and professionalism.

You can go http://medicalschoolhq.net/thankyous for several examples of email templates that you can use to craft your thank you notes.

I've used the word *email* several times to talk about sending thank you notes. It doesn't matter how you send them, but I prefer email because it's prompt and it goes directly to the computer of the person you are sending it to. In addition, I prefer email because some schools may not want you to send physical thank you notes to the school. They may have difficulty getting letters to the interviewers. If you are planning on sending physical thank you notes, double check with the school that it's okay to send them that way.

Another thing to keep in mind is that many schools will put your notes and any other correspondence in your file. Don't send the same exact email to every person or else it will look lazy on your part when they pull your file for review at a later time.

Remember: be prompt, include something unique from your discussions, and be respectful.

Debrief

Along with thank you notes, another time sensitive activity is to do a self-debrief. Use your pen and paper and write down what you think went right, and what you think went wrong. There is no better time than immediately after your interview when everything is fresh in your mind. Again, don't rely on your memory to retain this stuff—you will lose it.

Some things to think about include tricky questions that may have been asked by the interviewers, unique things about the campus that you did or didn't like, questions other students asked that you liked and hadn't thought of, and your overall impression of the school. Give it a rating from 1-10. Doing this will allow you to compare different schools when you get multiple acceptances. It will also help you learn from any mistakes you made so that for your next interview, you will be better prepared. Remember, according to Einstein, the definition of insanity is doing the same thing over and over again, but expecting a different result.

CHAPTER 9

COMMON MISTAKES

There are many reasons students fail to secure their acceptance on interview day. After successfully coaching students through the interview process and seeing the mistakes first hand, I was able to narrow down the list of mistakes to the seven mistakes I see most commonly. Remember, if you're at the interview, you have an opportunity, just like everybody else there, to get into that medical school. That medical school thoroughly vetted you up to that point; your grades are good enough, your MCAT scores are good enough, and your personal statement and your extracurricular activities are all good enough for you have an interview.

Interview spots are limited. They're a precious resource for that medical school, so there is a reason they are offering *you* an opportunity to interview. This day, the interview day, is your opportunity to show them the person behind the application, the letters of recommendation, your personal statement and extracurricular activities. They want to make sure that what they see on paper is who you are in person. That you can show up on time to the interview, dress appropriately, communicate clearly, express and feel empathy, and be friendly/respectful with/towards everyone—this is what they're looking for, and this is your opportunity to prove that.

Sounding Too Rehearsed

When you're asked a question, and it sounds like you're reading a script from the inside of your head, that's not good. This is supposed to be a conversation between you and your potential future colleague, and it's supposed to flow back and forth. It's not supposed to sound like you're regurgitating something that you've rehearsed over and over again. It doesn't come across as genuine.

A common problem that occurs when you have such a strict, scripted answer, is that if the interviewer can throw you off, or if you get interrupted somehow, you're going to falter because it's going to be difficult to find your place in that script. Don't get me wrong, you need to practice, and practice a lot, but you need to be able to intelligibly discuss and talk about everything that's going to come up during the interview. You need to know it all like you've rehearsed it 500 times, but you don't want it to sound like you memorized it.

You need to know it enough for you to be familiar with what the key points are, and with what the most important and relevant information is that you want to get across. You should be comfortable filling in the rest on the fly. That's how it should sound, and this is what you need to work on as you're preparing for your medical school interviews. Think about having lunch with a friend—do you go prepared with a script of all the answers to the questions he or she may ask you? No. You go in with one or two important things that you want to tell them, and you allow yourself to fill in the details as the conversation progresses.

One of the biggest and toughest questions that may be asked is the, "Tell me about yourself" question. It's a very easy, very open-ended question that interviewers may ask you because it tells them so much about you. It tells them about how you're able to open up a discussion, and put together your thoughts in an open-ended interview scenario. It can tell them about your values and about your ability to communicate. This is where I often see being too rehearsed come into play. We'll talk about this question more in-depth with actual responses from students in Section III of this book.

Inappropriate Appearance

This seems so simple and obvious that I shouldn't even have to mention it, but I do. This isn't something specifically related to the actual interview, but it does relate to your interview day.

You definitely want to be memorable during your interview day, but you don't want your clothes, makeup or hairstyle to be what's memorable about you.

I already covered what is appropriate in a previous chapter, so, if you have questions, please review that and follow that advice.

Answering Too Quickly or Interrupting the Interviewer

During the interview you may have a tendency to not fully pay attention to the full question the interviewer is asking because you're too busy formulating a response to the first part you've heard. When the interviewer is in the middle of asking a question, he or she may pause, and you may think that's your opportunity to jump in and start answering. Sometimes you may have the response ready, and you're excited to get it out because you've practiced it and rehearsed that specific answer ten times. The problem is that their pause might not be the time to start answering the question. Maybe they're pausing to consider how they're going to finish asking the question, or twist the question in some way.

Besides making sure that you're not interrupting the interviewer and answering the wrong question, make sure that you're taking the time to think through how you are going to answer the question. You need to take a pause after the interviewer asks the question. Ask yourself, "Did I understand what he or she just asked me?" If not, ask for clarification. If you need to pause for a bit longer because it's a hard question, or maybe because it's something that you haven't thought of before, go ahead and say, "That's something that I need to think about for a second." That's perfectly okay to do. Just sit there and think.

What you don't want to do is sit there in silence without asking for a second to think, or fill the dead air with verbal pauses like "um's" and "ah's." You also don't want to start to answer the question and then stop, and then start over, and then stop, and then start over. This can be perceived as not being able to comprehend, analyze, and answer the question. Take the time, take a pause—it's okay.

Going Off Topic

One of the things that happens, if you don't take that moment to pause and think about what was asked, is that you can go off topic. When you go off topic, you have the potential to start discussing topics not expected by the interviewer. You can fall into the trap of stretching your knowledge, and the interviewer can quickly catch on to this. They may try to follow up with more questions about your off topic rant to see how far you are willing to go before you admit that you are unsure of the points you are discussing. So answer what was asked of you, and no more. That's an easy way to stay safe.

Being Negative or Making Negative Statements

You should feel excited and positive to have the opportunity to be interviewed for a seat in the next medical school class. Unfortunately, students have a tendency of answering questions in a negative way, even if they don't intend to be negative.

If your interviewer asks you what your biggest challenge was with one of your grades, you may say, "You know what? That teacher, he was just terrible, and he had it out for the whole class. I did the best I could, but everybody failed, and he was just terrible." This is not the way to answer that question. If you did poorly in a class, you need to admit fault. If you got a C, a D, or an F, you obviously did something to contribute to earning that grade. Yes, even if the class was curved. When an interviewer is asking you a question based on a poor grade, they're looking to see who you place blame on and what your reaction to the situation is. As long as you accept the result, and talk about what you've learned from that situation, and how you are prepared to improve in the future, you're doing well. Again, you're at the interview, they have already vetted you and accepted that grade, you should too. Don't try to assign blame on other people, don't be negative about former bosses, classmates, or teachers. It's an easy trap to start answering a question and have negativity built into your response without you even realizing it.

During one of my mock interviews, I asked the student what the causes were of his less-than-stellar grades as he started his undergraduate career. He answered the question by saying he was unmotivated. That to me, as the interviewer, is a big red flag. That's a negative word that's describing this person, and it's a word that makes me worry that maybe he will fall back into an unmotivated state. The interviewer may follow up with questions to see what has changed so that you don't fall back into that old state.

After this mock interview, I brought up this point and said, "This is how you answered this question, and to me, that's a very negative way of answering it." We distilled down some more, and we talked about it more in-depth, and we found the core of him being unmotivated was the fact that he was distracted. He was distracted because he had to work to pay for his undergraduate education. He was distracted because he wanted to travel. He compressed a lot of classes into a shorter amount of time so that he could graduate early and do the traveling he was excited to do. Being distracted is a lot less negative than being unmotivated. I would argue that he was very motivated, just not for school work. He was motivated to finish early to travel, and he was motivated to pay for school. Using distraction, the true reason for his undergraduate performance, allows him to talk about what was distracting him and how those distractions are now behind him. I discussed earlier about how your life experiences are truly what separates you. This student's distractions hurt his grades but strengthened him as an applicant.

We did a follow-up interview, and I brought up the same question and asked him about his grades, and he said, "You know what? I was distracted during that time because of X, Y, Z, and here's what I learned from it."

This is how he answered the question during the actual interview, and it helped him earn an acceptance to medical school.

Not Smiling

There are some visual cues that make an interviewee be perceived as strong or not. If you don't smile, that's a big red flag. Again, this is supposed to be a conversation between you and your future colleague. How can you relax so that you are able to smile and answer questions in a conversational manner, regardless of how stressed-out you may be? Smiling, faked or not, has been proven to positively affect your mood. Even with a forced smile, you are happier. Happier people are friendlier and friendlier people are better conversationalists. Be happy!

Nervous Tics and Verbal Pauses

You need to understand what your nervous tics are, and if you use filler words like, "Um," "Uh" or "Ah." If you have some other gestures that you do that get in the way of effective communication and distract the interviewer from your interview responses and what you're actually saying, you need to be self-aware and willing to work on eliminating them. To accomplish this, you will need to do a video-recorded mock interview and get a video recording of how you respond so that you can see first-hand how those habits impact your ability to effectively communicate. At the bare minimum, you should have an audio recording so you can hear what your answers actually sound like. Ideally, you'll have a video recording so you can see how you react, see your nervous tics and anything else that may distract the interviewer.

On American Idol, Simon Cowell would often criticize a singer because of their facial expressions when they were singing. He said it distracted from their actual performance. It's the same for your medical school interview. Understand what you look like, so you can correct anything that may be distracting. With smartphones, we all carry video cameras in our pockets these days; prop it up on something and record away!

I had a student who I worked with who had a natural frown on her face. It was just the way her cheeks and lips lined up. There were times when she was talking that I thought she was sad. I mentioned this to her, and she had the ability to go back and watch. Over the next couple of interviews that we did together, she was able to consciously make an effort to smile, and the entire interview was much better. The whole dynamic of the interview changed because my perception of her changed and her energy levels were increased.

Not Having Proper Questions for the Interviewer

At the end of the interview, the interviewer is probably going to ask if you have any questions for him or her. You need to have good, solid, informed questions to ask. It shows that you're interested, that you've done your homework, that you're prepared, and that you care.

It allows you to build a deeper connection with the interviewer because you may ask a question they've never heard before. Or, you may ask a question and elicit a response or further a conversation with them that they're going to remember. And when they go back to the other admission committee members, they are more likely to speak on your behalf as to why you should have a seat at that medical school.

In the previous chapter, I covered how to prepare for asking the interviewer questions. It may be obvious, but I'll say it anyway: don't ask questions that you can find answers to with a simple search of the school's website. This shows laziness and a lack of caring. Have at least three questions ready to go for the interviewer.

Not Doing a Mock Interview

The biggest and costliest mistake that students make is not doing a mock interview with someone who they trust and who is intimately familiar with the interview process. The mock interview is the one place where you can work out the kinks so that you don't make any of the mistakes listed above on interview day.

The medical school interview is such a key part of the application process, but too many students take it for granted and think, "Well if I get an interview they obviously like my GPA, they like my MCAT, they like everything so they just want to make sure that I can talk." The majority of students probably don't do very well just by showing up and winging it during the interview.

The Admissions Committee is looking for so much more than that, so you need to understand and prepare for this. I hope this book helps you with some of that preparation. We'll cover more about the mock interview in a few chapters.

CHAPTER 10

HOW TO SUCCEED

The interview process isn't all doom and gloom! Obviously, there are several thousand students who start medical school each year after having successful interviews. The question is, what did they do to succeed?

Be Positive

The first step is to be positive. Have a positive attitude. Be confident in yourself. If that is not naturally who you are, then you need to fake it until you make it. Did you know that putting a pencil in your mouth to force a smile on your face makes you happier? Standing in a Wonder Woman pose for as little as two minutes also boosts your confidence and reduces stress hormones.

There is a great Ted Talk that I recommend you watch that covers these types of tricks. Go to Ted.com and search for 'Amy Cuddy: Your body language shapes who you are.'[10]

Eye Contact

You'd be surprised how little eye contact some students make during an interview. Remember, you are applying to medical school, to be a physician. When you are a physician, you need to interact with patients, families, colleagues and other healthcare professionals. Eye contact is a very important part of effective communication. If you're struggling with eye contact during an interview, how is the interviewer supposed to picture you interacting with a patient?

It's Okay to Have a Sense of Humor

During your interview, you need to be respectful, open and honest. You definitely need to believe in everything you are saying. Assume the interviewer is a human lie detector. Don't try to slide anything by him or her.

If you feel that the mood of the interview is right and there is an opportunity for humor, use it. The interviewer doesn't want dry discussions all day; a good laugh helps ease the tension. Don't overdo it, though!

Don't Argue

The interview is meant to test your personality, how you react and think. There may be times that the interviewer tries to draw you into an argument, or times where you may want to argue something the interviewer is saying. DON'T DO IT! I guarantee you that you will lose the argument and you will win a rejection letter at that medical school. It's not worth it.

Be Prepared

I've already covered how to prepare for your interview day. You need to know your application inside and out. You need to know the school, what they stand for, and why you want to go there. You need to know what is going on in the world of healthcare and beyond.

The best way to be prepared for your interview day is to do mock interviews. We'll cover that next.

CHAPTER 11

MOCK INTERVIEW PREP

I hope that after reading the first section of this book, you understand how important the medical school interview is. I don't care how much of a personality you think you have, or how well you think you communicate. Until you are placed in a room, sitting across from the person who controls whether or not you get into medical school, where your nerves can destroy your chances, you don't know anything.

Luckily, interview skills improve with practice—meaning the more you do, the better you'll get.

One strategy that others recommend, even though you don't have complete control over it, is to not schedule your first choice school as your first interview. You assume that this will give you a chance to *practice* at your other interviews.

However, there are a couple of major flaws in this approach. The first flaw is that you won't know until you are at the school and interacting with the students and faculty if you will truly love that school. Your first interview may have been at the bottom of your list, but after the interview day, you may be ready to move it to the top. So much for 'practice.'

The other major flaw in this approach is that you have absolutely no way of knowing how the interview went. You don't know if you answered questions well or if you rambled for 10 minutes. You'll go into subsequent interviews saying the same thing without any feedback on your previous interviews. Using Einstein's definition of insanity, going from interview to interview and expecting to get better without feedback is insane. This is not good practice for the interview.

So how do you get practice then? Your school's pre-health office likely has mock interview services that you can take advantage of, and I highly recommend that you use these services, rather than a general career counselor.

A general career counselor *may* be trained in medical school interviews, but I would use them as a last resort. The medical school interview is not a job interview. They are very different interviews with very different styles. I've worked with students who approach the interview like a job interview, and it doesn't end well.

You may be asking yourself "what is a mock interview?" Let's relate it to the MCAT. The majority of students who have taken the MCAT have taken practice tests. Those who don't take any practice tests probably shouldn't be applying because their score likely will not be very good. The mock interview is like an MCAT practice test. It familiarizes you with the process, but more importantly, it provides with you with vital feedback so that you can improve for the next time. That's all that the mock interview is—it's a practice test for your real interview. You will get dressed up, call in or go to an office, prepare questions and go through the interview like it's the real deal.

During the mock interview, you are recorded so that you can observe yourself from a more objective point of view. What are your nervous tics? What are your vocal pauses or filler words? What other gestures do you have? This is your opportunity to become self-aware and correct distracting behaviors. I do all of my mock interviews with students over Skype. I record the video and audio and upload the entire file so that each student can see and hear their performance soon after the interview is over.

The mock interview will probably be the first time that you actually say your answers out loud. In Section II of this book, there are over 575 questions to help you get an idea of what may be asked during your interview, but just thinking about the answer isn't good enough; it's very important to actually verbalize your answers. Until you say the words out loud, you don't know how they are going to sound, and you don't know how those words are going to land on someone else. Unfortunately, we always sound much better in our head than once we open our mouths. This is the key to the mock interview.

Once you have successfully completed a few mock interviews, you should have a good understanding of how well, or poorly, you will handle the stress of the actual interview day. After the mock interviews, you'll know how your body is going to respond. You'll know if you are going to freeze up in certain situations or become emotional in others. Going through a mock interview and receiving feedback is truly the best form of practice.

I've worked with both traditional and nontraditional students and helped them prepare for their interview day. I've worked with students applying for the first time, and students reapplying after failing during previous interviews. The goal is always the same—help students be the most prepared that they can be for their interview. Students I've worked with have been accepted and are now medical students at both MD and DO schools all across the country.

Just as you may see by working with well-trained advisors doing mock interviews, I have seen major transformations in students as they progress from the first interview to the last. You can see some of those transformations later in the book in Section III. These are transcripts from real interviews that I've done with students—their answers, and my feedback.

Please check out http://medicalschoolhq.net/mock-interview-prep/ for other ways in which I can help you prepare for your interview day.

SECTION II

THE QUESTIONS

CHAPTER 12

OPENING QUESTIONS

The opening of your interview can make or break you. The interviewer can start from a thousand different places, but listed here are a few of the more common places to start.

Remember that first impressions are made very quickly. Some business texts quote that a first impression is made within the first 7 seconds, while a psychology journal said it happens even faster than that—in 1/10th of a second[11]! Go in smiling, confident and ready to have a genuine conversation.

The goal with the opening question is to get through it and get to the next question. The goal of the next question is to get to the next. Take each question one at a time.

- Tell me about your early life.
- Assume that all of the information in your application is nonexistent (grades, activities, etc.). Tell me about yourself.
- Tell me your story.

- Why are you interested in this school?
- What have you enjoyed the most about today?
- Why medicine?
- Why do you want to be a doctor?

CHAPTER 13

GRADES AND MCAT SCORE QUESTIONS

A s noted in Section I, the interviewer may or may not have access to your academic records. In an open interview, although they will have access to this information, they may not look at it prior to the interview. In a closed (blind) or partially-blind interview, the interviewer won't have access to your scores beforehand.

The goal with these types of questions, as with every question, is to be honest and accept your shortcomings. If you did poorly, accept it. Own it. Don't place blame. Talk about what you learned and how you will move forward in the future, so you don't repeat the same mistakes.

- What was your GPA?
- What was your MCAT score?
- What do you think of your MCAT score?

- How did you go from a D to an A? What was your strategy? (assuming you repeated a class)
- Why are your two MCAT scores so different? (assuming you retook it)
- Your GPA is outstanding. Why is your MCAT score just average/below average?
- Why did you perform so poorly on [pick a section] of the MCAT?
- Explain the trends in your transcript.
- Explain this dip in your grades.
- Did you take an MCAT prep course?
- Did you have any academic difficulties in college?
- How did you overcome your academic difficulties?
- How much did you prepare for the MCAT?
- Why do you think you did so well on the MCAT?
- Why do you think you did poorly on the MCAT the first time you took it?
- Why did you take the MCAT so many times?
- Explain the grade you got in this class. (assuming it was less than stellar)
- Tell me about this [unusual] class that you took.
- Why did you choose to graduate from college in three years?
- Why did you do poorly during your first semester/year of college?
- What did you learn from doing poorly in that class?
- Medical school is much harder than undergrad. How are you going to avoid the academic difficulties that you struggled with previously?
- I see you struggled during your [pick a year/semester] in college. How can you reassure me that you are ready to handle medical school?
- Did you study for the MCAT (or a specific class) with a group of other students?
- Do you think doing well in undergrad will prepare you for medical school?

CHAPTER 14

EXTRACURRICULAR ACTIVITIES QUESTIONS

One of the biggest mistakes students make going into the interview is not reviewing every part of their application. This includes the extracurricular activities and the descriptions you wrote for each one, and which ones you labeled as most meaningful.

It is important to know your application inside and out. You need to understand your research and what was learned from it. You need to be able to talk about each of the experiences you included in your application. This is why it's important to only include the most meaningful experiences, instead of filling the space with items that don't add value or highlight your strengths.

- What was your most significant non-medically related volunteer activity?
- What was your most rewarding extracurricular activity?
- Why don't you have much shadowing experience?

- Describe your research to me as if I were a four-year-old.
- Describe your involvement in the [extracurricular activity].
- Describe your favorite patient interaction.
- What was your most memorable experience with [insert volunteer experience or travel]?
- Describe a time when you became close with a patient during your volunteer experiences.
- Describe a research experience that left a profound impression on you, and tell me what you learned from it.
- What activities do you participate in that are not work or school related?
- What has been your biggest leadership role?
- What has been your experience with the underserved population?
- Tell me about your ability to speak multiple languages.
- What sort of clinical experience have you received?
- How have your experiences made you want to pursue medicine?
- What is the hardest situation that you have encountered as a volunteer?
- Tell me about your mentoring experiences.
- Tell me about your travel experiences.
- Tell me about the music you play.
- How did your research change your outlook on medicine?
- How did you get involved in shadowing?
- What research/clinical experiences do you have?
- Tell me about a leadership experience.
- Tell me about your research.
- Why was your [insert extracurricular experience] so valuable to you?
- What do you do for fun?
- What are your activities and outlets outside of academics?
- Please describe your most significant life experience.
- What was the hardest situation you were in as a leader?

CHAPTER 15

"WHY MEDICINE?" QUESTIONS

I hope that if you have made to this stage of the application process and are preparing for interviews that you TRULY understand why it is that you want to become a doctor. It's not good enough to just want to help people, or to love science. It's not good enough to both love science AND want to help people. It's definitely not good enough to just love watching Grey's Anatomy. Dig deeper and be able to talk about what it is that is motivating you to be a physician.

- What was the process of elimination that led you to a career in medicine?
- Did your parents pressure you to go into medicine?
- Has anyone tried to convince you not to enter the medical profession?
- Did you ever waver in your decision to go into medicine?
- Did you ever consider any other professions?
- Did anyone push you to do medicine?
- What would you do with your life if medicine weren't an option?
- When did you decide medicine was your calling?

- Why not pursue becoming a PA/RN/NP?
- Why be a doctor and not a lawyer or business person?
- Why aren't you interested in an MD/PhD program?
- Have your parents influenced your decision to become a physician?
- Why do you want to undertake the MD/PhD dual degree?
- When did you first decide that you wanted to become a physician?
- How did [specific portion of essay] influence your decision to pursue [this type of] research?
- Why medical school?
- I see your parents are [another professional discipline i.e. dentists, physical therapists, etc.]. Why aren't you going into that profession?
- Why do you want to be a doctor?
- Why medicine?
- What was your 'a-ha' moment?
- What kind of doctor do you want to be?
- Being a doctor is harder than most careers, and you can make more money doing something else, so why are you doing this?
- What do you say to those physicians who are telling you not to pursue medicine?
- Is your mother or father a physician? If so, did he or she try to convince you not to pursue medicine?

CHAPTER 16

ETHICAL AND MORAL QUESTIONS

Ethical and moral questions seem to be one of the more stressful question types. But I want to tell you that with some good training, and the proper framework, these are actually the easiest!

The first question I typically get asked is if there is a right or wrong answer to ethical questions. The answer is NO; there is not. The interviewer is looking for your level of knowledge and your ability to think about the subject on a level higher than just yourself. You need to always look at both sides of the situation, respect both sides, but ultimately pick a side. If you are asked to assert a point of view, but can't, that shows the interviewer that there is a potential lack of decision-making skills.

These questions are often times meant to take you out of your comfort zone, so you need to be prepared to handle that. These aren't common dinner table conversations, so it's likely you haven't really had a dialog about these topics before. A good strategy is to think out loud while answering the question, which will help the interviewer understand your thinking, and allow them to hear your decision-making process. It is important that you always remain respectful of the side that you ultimately don't support. Being rude or condescending in this situation is the wrong move.

If you responded to a question about abortion with: "I think anybody who has an abortion should go to jail. I'm pro-life and wouldn't perform abortions on anybody and would question the judgment of physicians who do." Here, you jumped to one side and didn't give any consideration of the other perspective. You also didn't give any thought to the patient. This is not good! You need to say something more respectful, like this: "I understand that there are some people who need abortions for health purposes, and those who get them for other reasons, but I personally would not perform them. I'd make sure that the patient's needs were met and would find them a physician to perform the procedure if that's what the patient ultimately wanted." In this second statement you were still able to stick to your guns, but you kept the patient's needs/wishes ahead of your personal agenda.

For every question asked, the patient's needs and safety should come first. Be respectful of both sides of the debate. Be confident in your decision and the side that you support.

- How would you deal with a colleague/patient who had different values/ beliefs than you?
- What would you do if your boss made an error and tried to hide it?
- What would you do if you saw your best friend cheating on a test in medical school?
- If you're in a car accident with a driver who you know is HIV-positive, and he needs first aid, would you help him knowing that you don't have any protective equipment?
- Is it ever ethical to lie to a patient?
- What would you do if a friend or colleague had a problem with alcohol or drug use?
- What would you do if a patient came to you and asked you to perform a procedure that you absolutely refuse to do?
- If you know your colleague was lying to patients, what would you do?

- What would you do if a doctor showed up to work with alcohol on her breath?
- Does it matter if a doctor who shows up to work with alcohol on his breath is a surgeon or primary care doctor?
- How would you treat a patient who refuses a blood transfusion based on religious beliefs?
- What do you think of the #BlackLivesMatter movement?
- What are your thoughts on abortion?
- Should we have the death penalty?
- What would you do if you were treating an eight-year-old child who was in a car accident and needed surgery and a blood transfusion, but the parents were Jehovah's witnesses?
- An alcoholic and a non-alcoholic need a liver transplant. There is only one liver to give. How do you choose who gets it?
- Two people need lung transplants today, or they will die. There is one lung available. One person smokes, and one person doesn't. How do you choose who gets the lung? What if the smoker has been on the transplant list for three times as long as the non-smoker?
- If someone gave you concert tickets to see your favorite band play, and you knew the tickets were stolen, would you still go?
- Do you think we should keep people alive for as long as we do on machines, knowing that the majority of our healthcare dollars are spent treating patients at the end of life?
- Can you be religious without being ethical?
- Describe an ethical dilemma and how you resolved it.
- Do you believe physicians have to be 100% honest with their patients?
- Do you believe that physicians ought to be upstanding citizens in the community?
- Do you think friends/family members should be allowed to donate organs to relatives who are not number one on the donor recipient list?
- Do you think people should be able to pay for organs if people are willing to sell them?

- A patient on whom you did a vasectomy comes in to have it redone because his wife is pregnant. You start the procedure and realize the vasectomy is intact, and there is no way your patient got his wife pregnant. What do you do?
- What are your thoughts about the stories of doctors and nurses cutting off life support to those stranded by Hurricane Katrina?
- A patient who has previously declined blood transfusions for religious purposes is now unconscious. Would you give them the transfusion now?
- You are the physician who has final authority for an insurance company. How do you tell another physician that the policy for their 20-year-old patient won't continue to cover life support?
- What would you do if your patient's family asked you to not disclose his terminal cancer diagnosis for fear that it would cause tremendous psychological harm?
- If all of your options are exhausted, and your patient is dying of a terminal illness and is in a lot of pain and already on maximum amounts of morphine, would you order more, knowing that it will likely kill him?
- Your patient contracted HIV from an affair. He refuses to tell his wife. What do you do?
- Should parents be allowed to clone their dying child?
- Would you tell a patient that you made a mistake, even if there were no consequences of that mistake?
- Do you think we should be allowed to give patients placebo treatments?
- Do you think it's moral for pharmaceutical companies to charge so much for medications?
- Do you think it's okay to use animals for research?
- If you had a limited supply of drugs, how do you decide which patients will get them?
- If you had suspicions that your research mentor or principal investigator was manipulating data, what would you do?

- The attending surgeon shows up for surgery drunk, and no one intervenes. What do you do? Does it matter if you're a premed, medical student, or resident?
- If we were to believe in the survival of the fittest theory, why should we waste resources saving those at the end of life?
- Would you perform an abortion?
- What would you do if you were asked to perform a procedure that you disagreed with for non-medical reasons?
- Do you think we should provide healthcare for illegal immigrants?
- Would you prescribe painkillers to a patient claiming to be in pain, even if you can't find any physical reasons for the pain on exam?
- Do you think we should have to opt-out of organ donation versus opt-in?
- Do you think gender reassignment surgery should be covered by insurance?
- I'm the father of a child who died because you accidentally gave him the wrong medication. What would you say to me?
- What do you tell the parents of your patient who are refusing vaccinations for their child?
- If you were a pediatrician, would you see patients whose parents refuse vaccines?
- What do you know about stem cell research?
- With people like Bill Gates and Mark Zuckerberg donating a lot of money to science, do you think it's ethical that these wealthy individuals dictate which diseases and organizations receive the most money?
- It's the end of your ED shift, and you have tickets to the opera. A patient is urgently rolled in in cardiac arrest. You see your replacement, but she's at least a minute out. What do you do?
- Do you think drugs like HGH and testosterone should be more readily available for aging men?
- Do you think illicit drugs should be legal?
- It seems like alcohol does more damage to our society than any other illicit drug. Should alcohol be illegal for everyone?

CHAPTER 17

POLITICS, POLICY AND HEALTHCARE QUESTIONS

ere is where we get into the nitty-gritty of healthcare. As I talked about earlier, it is important that you to stay up-to-date with what is going on in the world around healthcare. This includes reading the news, popular websites and books surrounding the career you are preparing to enter.

I'll often get into discussions with students about the Affordable Care Act, or our healthcare system as a whole. It floors me when some students have no idea what they are getting themselves into. How can you plan on spending 7+ years of your life and several hundred thousand dollars to join a profession that you know little about outside of shadowing and some clinical experience?

Stay informed so you can discuss any of these topics with your interviewer.

Concierge Medicine is becoming an increasingly popular option for physicians. How do you feel about this, and what are the consequences of this practice?

- If you've been given a magic wand to fix any problem in the world, which problem would you tackle?
- What is the hardest thing about being a patient?
- What is the hardest thing about being a doctor?
- Studies show that only 6% of Americans engage in all five of the health behaviors known to reduce chronic disease. How do you fix that?
- Do you know what the five health behaviors are for reducing chronic disease?
- If you're trying to prove that stem cell research is worth funding, what types of experts would you seek out?
- What do you think is the greatest challenge for doctors?
- How do you think the healthcare system can be fixed?
- What do you think is the greatest accomplishment in healthcare in the last 20 years?
- What role does the physician have in educating patients about health in general?
- Describe a challenge in healthcare today and a way to solve it.
- What has your [family member who is a physician] told you about medicine?
- Why do you think drug and alcohol abuse rates are high among physicians?
- Tell me about some of your political views.
- How would you reduce costs of medicine?
- What are your thoughts on HMOs?
- As a physician how will you deal with your mistakes?
- What is the biggest problem facing medicine today?
- Do you think healthcare is a human right?
- What are your thoughts on the Affordable Care Act?
- What are the pros of the Affordable Care Act?
- What are the cons of the Affordable Care Act?

- If you were in charge, how would you fix healthcare?
- Do you think doctors are paid fairly?
- Do you think we should have universal healthcare?
- Why do you think physicians complain about reimbursement rates, considering being a physician is one of the most well-paid careers?
- Can you compare the healthcare system in the U.S. to that in Canada?
- What do you think of when you hear patient-physician relationship?
- How did the U.S. rank in the last World Health Organization rankings of healthcare systems?
- Why do you think the U.S. healthcare system was ranked so low in the last World Health Organization rankings?
- Define HMO.
- Define Medicare.
- Define Medicaid.
- Define PPO.
- How do you feel that healthcare is working in the United States?
- How do you think the problem of rising medical costs can be solved?
- Describe some of the problems in healthcare that are most troubling to you.
- Describe the qualities which make a physician a good leader.
- How would you handle a patient who does not take his or her medications or show up to office visits?
- How would you solve the problem of the uninsured/underinsured?
- How do you feel about poverty in America?
- What would be your biggest fear in practicing medicine?
- Discuss a healthcare issue which has been in the news in the past month.
- Do nurses who obtain PhDs have the right to call themselves Doctor in a clinical setting?
- What role do you think the pharmaceutical industry should have in medical education?
- What do you think about the VA system replacing physician anesthesiologists with CRNAs?

- Do you think that pharmaceutical companies should be able to advertise directly to consumers? Why or why not?
- What is the percentage of uninsured persons in the U.S.?
- What would be some of the things that you would consider in treating a patient who is in chronic pain?
- Do you think it is important for a physician to be humble?
- Do you think women and men have equal opportunities as practicing physicians?
- What would you do with a noncompliant patient?
- What do you think about the surgical residency program that told one of its residents to not return to the program after becoming paraplegic?
- What do you think is going to happen to healthcare in the future?
- What do you think about alternative medicine?
- What worries you about healthcare?
- What do you think about telemedicine?
- Where do you think the Supreme Court is heading?
- How would you deal with the drug problem in the world?
- Should funding for research only be given to projects with immediate direct clinical applications, or all projects which seek to understand the world around us?
- With alternative medicine becoming more popular, how do you see your role as a physician integrating this practice with Western medicine?
- If a medication in a trial has shown good results with no major side effects, should the FDA approve it for those patients for whom waiting would lead to death or worsening quality of life, without going through the normal process that medications go through?
- Why do you think there is so much burnout among physicians?
- How do you think we can help the underserved and uninsured afford health insurance?
- What is your opinion on the current state of the U.S. healthcare system?
- Do you think we'll ever cure cancer?
- What do other countries do better than we do in healthcare? Why?
- How would you fix our obesity epidemic?

- How can the medical system be fixed to allow equal healthcare access?
- Do you think it's fair that physicians can get sued for bad outcomes?
- Do you think physicians should be barred from being able to go on strike?
- Do you think every state should have the same healthcare plans?
- What three changes in the delivery of healthcare would you like to see?
- How would you solve the tremendous organ supply shortage for organ donation programs?
- What would you like to see implemented in healthcare policy by the government?
- Do you think raising minimum wage is a solution to the inequalities in the U.S.?
- Do you think it's important to stress the use of preventive medicine to patients?
- How do you stress the importance of preventive medicine to patients?
- Do you think physicians should be rewarded if they don't order a lot of tests?
- Name the three diseases/conditions responsible for the most deaths in the U.S. per year.
- What do you think about the war on terrorism?
- Do you think the British or American medical system is better?
- Do you think we should put extra taxes on junk food and soda?
- How would you convince a teenager to stop smoking?
- Are PAs relevant?
- What do you think about gay marriage?
- In an affluent country like the United States, why is healthcare still so hard for people to access?
- How would you explain our healthcare system to someone from Canada?
- Do you think antibiotics should be more regulated to help prevent resistant bacteria?
- What needs to be addressed in medicine in the next ten years?
- What is the biggest challenge for physicians in the next ten years?

- Do you think nutrition education is something which should be included in medical school curriculums?
- How much of a role do you think nutrition plays in a person's disease/condition?

CHAPTER 18

'YOUR FUTURE' QUESTIONS

Questions about your future give the interviewer some insight into how much you've thought about being a physician. Women often joke that they've envisioned their wedding ceremony since they were young girls. Questions about your future show the interviewer that you've been thinking about this more than just a last second decision to apply.

Questions about your future can include scenarios about where you are practicing, what type of medicine you're practicing, your general approach to the medical field and your long-term goals. Be prepared to talk about challenges with the healthcare system, just like in the healthcare section before this.

- What would you do instead of medicine?
- What do you want to do after medical school?
- How will you balance the time to do research and see patients?
- What do you want to do once you are done with your MD/PhD training?
- How do you plan to incorporate your MPH into your medical career?

- What are your 15-year goals?
- Do you see yourself in academic medicine or private practice?
- After medical school and residency, perhaps 7-12 years down the road, where do you see yourself?
- Fifteen years from now, what do you see as being your toughest challenge?
- What is your dream situation ten years from now?
- Are there any areas of medicine which interest you more than others?
- Are you considering an MPH?
- Are you interested in [insert specialty] because of your research experience?
- Are you interested in pursuing [insert specialty]?
- Are you planning on staying in [insert state/city] after graduation?
- What are your future career plans?
- How do you see yourself redefining medicine in the course of your career?
- Are you interested in academic medicine?
- What sort of difficulties do you expect to face in medical school?
- Do you plan to do research during your career as a doctor?
- How do you want to contribute to medicine?
- Do you think you'll practice what you preach as a physician?
- Do you want to work in an underserved community?
- What impact do you want to make on the field of medicine?
- At the end of your career, how will you determine if you had a successful career?
- What will you do if you realize, five years into practice, that you don't like medicine?
- Do you see yourself as treating sick people or healthy people?
- What will you want your medical school classmates to remember you for in 20 years?
- How do you expect to change in medical school?
- When you are 65, and you are looking back at your life, what do you want to be able to tell your grandkids?

CHAPTER 19

PERSONAL QUESTIONS

I hope I've stressed it enough up to this point that you are being interviewed because the school wants to know more about *you*. The questions in this section help the interviewer learn more about you as a person, including your likes and dislikes, and your strengths and weaknesses.

In the "Before the Interview" chapter, I mentioned the importance of asking friends and family for input. This is where all that input gets put to good use.

- What was the last movie that you saw?
- What is the last book that you read?
- What do you like to do in your spare time?
- What was your favorite class?
- What would you want your patients to say about you?
- What was your hardest class in college?
- Why would you want to stay in [insert state/city] after being here so long?
- How would your friends describe you?

- I'm visiting your state, and I've never been there before. Where would you take me?
- What are your weaknesses?
- What are your hobbies?
- What do you do to relax?
- What do you like about the city where you're from?
- What has been your greatest challenge?
- What is on your nightstand?
- What is on your bookshelf?
- What station is your TV tuned to when it's turned on?
- What is on your MP3 player?
- How have you experienced working in a group?
- Tell me about a time when you worked in a group, and it did not work out well.
- Tell me about a time when you worked in a group, and it worked out very well.
- If you had to choose between pursuing the MD or the PhD degree only, which would you choose and why?
- What are three adjectives you would use to describe yourself?
- Discuss a time you showed compassion.
- Discuss a time you needed help.
- What personal characteristics do you have that will make you a good fit for a career in medicine?
- What would your obituary say?
- How would your best friend describe you?
- What non-academic book have you read recently?
- What do you like to do for fun?
- What qualities will you bring to the medical school class?
- Are you worried about the transition to medical school?
- What is a sacrifice that you made for someone else?
- What role would you play in a group scenario trying to solve a problem?
- Tell me about your family.

- Talk to me about your experience with [condition/disease that you've written about in an essay].
- Who in your family has had the most influence on you?
- Tell me more about your neighborhood as a child.
- What are you doing now that you are out of school? (assuming you're a nontraditional student or have taken a gap year)
- What are you passionate about?
- What have you discovered through your research?
- Have you had any extraordinary challenges or difficulties growing up?
- What was the most challenging part about living in [state/city/country]?
- Do you have any pets?
- Tell me about your siblings.
- Are there any physicians in your family?
- Are there any other healthcare professionals in your family? (dentists, PAs, physical therapists, etc.)
- Are you a group leader?
- Are you a leader or a follower?
- Do you like music?
- Are you a problem-based learning or traditional lecture type of learner?
- Are you a perfectionist?
- How does your perfectionism affect your ability to work in groups?
- Do you expect perfection from others?
- Are you a risk-taker?
- Are you an activist?
- Are you arrogant?
- Have you faced any hardships in your life?
- Why did you choose your undergraduate school?
- Have you ever had someone close to you struggle with substance abuse? If so, how did you help him or her?
- Who shaped who you are today?
- At your funeral, what would you want people to say about you?
- How has your time off from school helped you as an applicant?
- Why did you take a gap year?

- How do you feel your previous career will help you as a physician? (assuming you're a nontraditional student)
- What is your biggest weakness?
- Tell me about a time when you failed. What was the result?
- Tell me about a time when you did something wrong. What happened?
- What would a friend say bugs him the most about you?
- What would your parents say is your biggest weakness?
- What would your friends say is your greatest strength?
- Can you think of a time when you disagreed with someone but decided to yield to their point of view?
- What was your hometown like?
- Could you describe yourself in a tweet? (140 characters or less)
- Describe yourself in one word.
- Tell me about a negative situation that you turned into a positive.
- Describe a creative project that you were involved with or a time when you showed leadership in a project or a program.
- Describe a difficult situation that you faced. What values and resources did you call on to make it through?
- Describe a difficult time and what you did to overcome it.
- Describe a positive learning experience.
- Describe a situation in which your interpersonal skills helped accomplish a goal.
- Describe a situation in which you went above and beyond.
- Describe a time in which you failed at something. (does not have to be academic)
- Describe a time when you needed to ask for help.
- Describe a time when you were misjudged.
- Describe something you regret.
- Describe yourself in a Snapchat Snap. (10 seconds)
- Describe a typical day for you.
- Describe one particularly difficult day that you had at school.
- Describe an experience working in small groups.
- Describe the biggest obstacle in your life.

- What is your biggest source of motivation and support?
- What makes you unique?
- Describe your greatest accomplishment.
- Describe your ideal mentor.
- Describe your support system.
- Describe yourself in three words.
- Do you consider yourself disadvantaged in any way?
- Do you like to spend time alone?
- What do you think about when you're alone?
- Do you rely on your parents for advice when facing a significant problem?
- Who do you rely on for advice?
- How will you handle being with students who are much younger than you? (assuming you're a nontraditional student)
- Tell me about a time you were misjudged.
- Have you ever been misunderstood?
- Describe a situation in which you did something that you truly regretted?
- How would you contribute to the diversity of the next class?
- What would the people you work with change about you?
- If you could change one thing about yourself, what would it be?
- Why are you changing careers mid-life to become a physician? (assuming you're a nontraditional student)
- What drives you?
- How do you take criticism?
- Why are the students in your class going to value you as a classmate?
- What is an unsolvable problem that you have faced in life?
- What attributes would you bring to a small group?
- How do you see your religion factoring into your decision-making in medicine? (assuming you're religious)
- What is your worst quality?
- Tell me about the criminal charges on your record. (assuming you have a criminal record)
- What will be hardest for you to sacrifice as a medical student?
- What will be hardest for you to sacrifice as a physician?

- What will be the biggest challenge for you as a medical student next year?

CHAPTER 20

SCHOOL RELATED QUESTIONS

Medical schools know that you probably didn't apply to just their school, and they aren't mad at you for that. What they will be unhappy with is if you don't know why you applied to their school. The school wants to make sure that you will be happy with your decision to go there. You need to do your research and determine the specific reason for applying to each school. We discussed this research in the "Before the Interview" chapter.

Below are the questions that an interviewer may ask you to dig deeper into your reasons.

- What other medical schools have you applied to?
- Why [insert school name]?
- What does [insert school name] have to offer you?
- Why should [insert school name] accept you?
- What made you want to come to [insert school name] since you're originally from [insert city/state]?

- What department do you see yourself joining if accepted to the [insert school name] MD/PhD program?
- If you were in my shoes and you had to present your case to the rest of the Admissions Committee, what would you want to say to them?
- What are you looking for in a school?
- After being in the North for so long, why do you want to come down South?
- Do you have any reservations about coming here?
- Could you handle our winters? (assuming you're from a warm place)
- Are you comfortable working with a patient base that is mostly made up of African-Americans and people of varying socioeconomic backgrounds?
- Are you concerned about making the transition from a small liberal arts college to a big university?
- Are you ready for the curriculum we have?
- Assuming that you are accepted to all schools at which you've interviewed, what's the most important factor in choosing a school?
- Did you apply to other schools around here?
- Why are you applying to just MD programs since you are also applying to MD/PhD programs?
- Do you think you're a better applicant than the others who are interviewing today?
- How do you feel about entering school while the curriculum is undergoing changes?
- How do you feel about our status of not being fully accredited? (for new medical schools)
- Are we your top choice?
- What are your considerations when deciding which school to attend?
- If you were accepted by all of the schools you applied to, would you come here?
- Which faculty members here are you considering working with? (usually an MD/PhD question)

CHAPTER 21

MISCELLANEOUS QUESTIONS

This last set of questions is the catch-all for questions that don't really fit in the other categories. That doesn't mean these aren't as important as the other sections, so pay as much attention to this section as the others.

- Are you sure you'll be able to handle the rigor of the basic science years? (assuming you're a non-science major or a nontraditional student)
- I read [insert story] in your secondary. Tell me more about it.
- Are there any red flags in your application that I should know about?
- Do you have any regrets about the major that you chose?
- Why did you choose your major?
- What can you bring to the profession of medicine?
- As your advocate on the Admissions Committee, what would you like me to stress about you as an applicant?

- As a physician, you might have to face very difficult situations in which your first plan of action fails. How has your background prepared you to face failure as a physician?
- What do you suggest that I should look for in an applicant?
- What would you tell the Admissions Committee about why you should be admitted over someone else?
- Tell me about Dr. [insert name] and why you think he/she wrote a letter of recommendation for you.
- Is there anything else that you want me to tell the committee?
- What is not in your file that you would like me to tell the committee?
- How would you want me to describe you to the Admissions Committee?
- Can you describe a non-science class that you have taken that stood out to you?
- Did you enjoy taking humanities classes along with your science classes?
- What was your favorite non-science class?
- You have 2 minutes to convince me to choose you over other applicants. Go!
- What was the most interesting class that you took in college?
- How did you get from an undergrad major in [insert major] to medicine?
- How did you decide which college to attend for undergrad?
- Can you explain the gap in your undergrad education?
- What on your application are you most proud of?
- If you had to work with someone whose personal beliefs were vastly different than yours and it caused problems at work, what would you do?
- What would you like me to write about you in your evaluation?
- What would you change about your college experience?
- Why did you go to [insert college]?
- Name two people, dead or alive, who you would like to meet and have dinner with.
- What would you do to ensure good communication between yourself and your colleagues?
- What would you define as the top 3 qualities of the perfect physician?

- Name a time when you went above and beyond and what you learned from the experience.
- Tell me about a time when you dealt with a problem, and what did you do?
- Do you watch CNN or Fox News?
- What qualities do you want in a physician who treats your family members?
- How would you explain to a two-year-old how to brush her teeth?
- What are the top 6 medical discoveries of all time?
- What makes you think you can handle the rigors of medical school?
- Were the premed students at your undergrad institution competitive?
- Is there anything you were hoping we'd talk about that hasn't been brought up yet?
- What can I tell you about [this city] and [this school]?
- Is there any info not on your application that you want to add?
- Tell me about the most interesting patient that you've seen.
- Is there anything that you want to tell me that might not be in your file?
- Is there anything that you would like to highlight about yourself that is not covered in your application?
- Are you comfortable with your own mortality?
- Are you prepared for the time commitment, financial burden, and hard work involved in an MD (or MD/PhD) program?
- What's the best piece of advice that you have been given?
- If you could travel back in time to have lunch with someone, who would it be?
- Can you give me a book recommendation?
- Can you think of a physician in your life who has stood out to you?
- Define curiosity.
- Define humanism.
- Tell me about the greatest challenge that a leader faces.
- Define integrity.
- Define professionalism.
- What does the term doctor-patient relationship mean to you?
- What do you anticipate will be the most difficult part of medical school?

- Describe what a leader is.
- What do you think makes a great leader?
- What book have you read that has impacted the way you think?
- Describe your legacy as you would like it to be 40 years from now.
- Describe your perfect day in which you could go anywhere with anyone and do anything.
- Do you have a medical role model?
- Do you have any biases?
- What do you think the word community means?
- Do you think research is something medical students should be required to do?
- Do you prefer to be a leader or follower?
- What is your ideal learning style?
- Who is your favorite author?
- Where do you get your news from?
- Tell me what you don't like about research.
- What is the best thing that you have done for another person?
- You just found out that your pregnant patient will have a child with [insert genetic condition]. Break the news to me as if I'm the patient.
- Do you think morality is genetic?
- Do you think empathy is genetic?
- Define bedside manner.
- How do you think your relationship with your parents will influence your bedside manner?
- What is the role of religion in medicine?
- Where were you on 9/11?
- If you could wave a magic wand and change anything about the world, what would you change?
- What is the most important trait in a doctor?
- I'm a nine-year-old patient and you are my Pediatric Oncologist. Explain to me my new diagnosis of terminal cancer.
- Do you know what it's like to be sick, or to be a patient?
- What do you value most in your friends?

- Marvel Comics or DC Comics?
- Who is your hero?
- Who would win, Batman or Superman?
- What role will you play in this class if accepted?
- What does love mean to you?
- What is a more important trait as a physician, compassion or intelligence?
- What would you do to reduce physician suicide rates?
- What technology will have the biggest impact on healthcare in the next 10 years?
- What makes you laugh?
- If you were in my shoes, what question would you ask yourself?
- What are some things that you'd change about the way your mom or dad practiced medicine, and some things that you'd keep the same? (assuming your mom or dad is a physician)
- If you had a family event that conflicted with patient care, how do you decide what is most important?
- What is a newspaper article that you read recently that disturbed you?
- Do you have any hesitations about attending medical school?
- What makes you special?
- What is something that no one else knows about you?
- Knowing you will have patients die or not respond to treatment, how will you deal with this?
- What would you be willing to do to get into medical school?
- Do you think that people can change themselves for other people?
- What is it that has allowed you to accomplish so much in your life?
- Do you think technology should replace human cadavers in anatomy lab?
- I'm not convinced that you've shown a sufficient interest in medicine. Convince me.
- Do you think countries should have borders?
- Do you think it's fair that a person's fate is often determined solely by where they were born?
- Do you think that we should have a wall preventing immigrants from entering the U.S.?

- Who is your favorite superhero? Why?
- Did you change your social media accounts before you applied so a school couldn't find you?
- What is social media's role in healthcare?
- What should be done in the educational system in the U.S. to motivate and retain underachieving students?
- If a physician who is perceived to be a great doctor abuses his family at home, should he still be allowed to practice medicine?
- Who is your favorite U.S. president and why?
- How would you explain to a five-year-old girl how to tie her shoelaces?
- Describe your apartment.
- What movie should all premed students watch?
- What book should all premed students read?
- Tell me about a day that you wish you could relive?
- Which of your letter writers knows you best?
- Have you ever known any bad doctors?
- What is society's biggest problem?
- How would you diffuse a situation with a hostile patient?
- How will you manage medical school with your family responsibilities? (assuming you have a family that you are responsible for)
- How will you ensure that you don't become jaded during your medical education?
- Why do you think the majority of physicians report they are burnt out on surveys?
- Why will you make a good doctor?
- What qualities in a person should make them not pursue becoming a physician?
- Is it fair for people to be judged based on first impressions?
- How do you think your parent's death will impact you as a physician? (assuming you have experienced the loss of a parent)
- Why should we reject you?
- Assuming we eventually colonize Mars, would you want to live there?

- If you could only do one, MD or PhD, which would you choose and why? (assuming you are applying to a dual-degree program)
- How do you know when to ask for help and when to do something on your own?
- Do you think it's okay to cry with, or in front of, a patient?
- How do you know when you've done enough?
- What was the worst day of your life?
- What hobby would you like to continue the most during medical school?
- Why did it take you so long to decide to change careers and go into medicine? (assuming you're a nontraditional student)
- Would you give your telephone number out to patients?
- As a woman, how do you plan on balancing a career with having a family?
- What is your favorite color?
- What is your favorite food?
- What is your favorite sport?
- What is missing from good patient care?
- Do you think physicians are more important than other members of the healthcare team?
- What would you do to end world hunger?
- What would you do to end violence in the world?
- What would you do to end world poverty?
- Define emotional maturity.
- Which book character best represents you?
- Which book character would you like to have dinner with?
- What's the difference between a good premed student and a bad one?
- What's more important for a physician, integrity or compassion?
- When was the last time you cried?
- Which third year rotation are you looking forward to the most?
- Do you think a physician's appearance matters to the patient?
- What is the role of the white coat?
- What era or time period would you want to live in?
- If we ranked all the students interviewing today, where would you rank?

- Do you think torture is justified to help protect our country?
- Do you think students who come from a family of physicians have an advantage?
- What is your favorite medical TV show?
- Tell me about a negative character trait and how would you deal with this in a patient.
- If you could be any animal, which would you be and why?
- If you could be any human organ, which would you be and why?
- Who would you bring on a road trip?
- What would you do if you had 24 hours to live and could go anywhere in the world?
- How does your family feel about your accomplishments?
- Do you think professional athletes are overvalued in our society?
- You interviewed here last year—what has changed since then?
- You applied here last year but weren't offered an interview. What have you done to improve your application?
- How is your relationship with your siblings? (assuming you have siblings)
- Do you think a surgeon needs to have an ego?
- Would you legalize marijuana on a federal level?
- Why do doctors need compassion?
- What qualities do you possess that will make you a great physician?
- What superpower would you like to have?

CHAPTER 22

MULTIPLE MINI INTERVIEW SCENARIOS

The Multiple Mini Interview (MMI), as we talked about earlier, operates with multiple stations that you will rotate through during your interview day. Each station will present you with a different scenario to work through with the interviewer or with an actor while the interviewer is observing you.

Let's talk about a specific scenario that you may encounter and what some of the background information may be that you won't know about.

Scenario: You are leaving work, and as you back out of your space, you hit another car without realizing it. The next day your boss asks you to come to her office.

Your boss is in the room

The Instructions for the Interviewer as the observer:

History: The car you hit was your boss' new Porsche that she bought last week. Your boss was excited to buy the Porsche because it reminded her of driving around in her dad's Porsche when she was a kid. It was the 10th anniversary of her dad's death last week, and she bought the car to remember him by. Having her new car damaged she takes as a reflection of the relationship she had with him, which wasn't always the best.

Focus: This station is intended to allow the observer to evaluate the applicant's communication skills. The actor will react and take cues from the applicant, but should try to remain as standard as possible across all students.

The sample MMI scenarios below are just a sample of what you might expect.

As the student, you will only be given the scenario, but the interviewer will know the background as to why the actor is acting the way they are.

The interviewer will be given a list of communication skills that you may be displaying. These would include being apologetic, listening well, being supportive, not dismissing your boss' concerns, and assuring your boss that her feelings are normal and reasonable.

As you read the scenario, try to think about the background behind the scenario. Try to think about what may be going on in the life of the other person. This helps you maintain an open mind when you enter the room and are faced with an angry actor. Thinking about what they may be going through will allow you to dig deeper with the questions you may ask. Remember to listen, especially to the scenarios with actors. I like the saying that you were given two ears and one mouth for a reason—to listen twice as much as you speak. The better you are at listening, the better your responses will be. The actor will likely try to lead you to certain questions based on their response.

When you are dealing directly with the interviewer, and you need to discuss some ethics behind a scenario, remember that there is no right or wrong answer. You are being tested on your ability to give your thoughts and ideas clearly, and to stand behind them if they are challenged.

The other thing to think about when you are reading the scenario is what kind of follow-up questions may be asked. For instance, if the topic of healthcare comes up, you may be asked about the Affordable Care Act, single payer healthcare systems, how to control healthcare costs, etc. If you are put in a scenario of a coworker stressed about paying bills, you may be asked about the cost of medical education, or when you would report a coworker to your superiors or the state licensing board.

Here are some more scenarios to think about:

SCENARIO 1

Prompt for Student

You and Emily, one of your best friends, are supposed to fly to Minnesota for a wedding. You go to pick up Emily at her house. **Emily is in the room.**

Background Information Given to the Evaluator/ Interviewer

Even though Emily is one of your best friends, you don't know that she is terrified of flying. It has never come up before because she hasn't flown since she was in high school, long before you met her. When you walk into the room, you can immediately tell that she has been crying and she looks very scared.

SCENARIO 2

Prompt for Student

Your co-worker, Dr. Smith, seems to be very negative about his patients lately. He recently joked about prescribing homeopathic medications to his patients who continue to complain of symptoms despite completely normal testing. He made it clear that he doesn't think these medications work, but he needs to give the patients something so that they will leave him alone. **Dr. Smith is in the room. Enter the room and discuss your concern that he is prescribing medications that don't work, and discuss his negative attitude towards his patients.**

Background Information Given to the Evaluator/Interviewer

Dr. Smith has been practicing medicine for five years, and he is burned out. He went to medical school because his parents really wanted him to be a physician. He is feeling unfulfilled and frustrated by patients who don't seem to have anything wrong with them. He's been thinking about quitting recently and looking for the right time.

SCENARIO 3

Prompt for Student

One of your co-workers, a surgeon, let it slip that his vision is deteriorating from a rare eye condition that will likely leave him blind. He has two kids and a wife who stays at home. He has told you that he doesn't plan on telling his employer because he needs to work and pay off his student loans and other bills. **What concerns do you have, and how would you go about helping your friend? Enter the room and discuss with the interviewer.**

SCENARIO 4

Prompt for Student

You are a pediatrician and notice that there are suspicious bruises on one of your regular patients. You've heard rumors of the father being an alcoholic who is sometimes abusive. The patient, mother, and father are in the room with you. **Consider how you would have a discussion with the patient and/or parents in this situation. Enter the room and discuss with the interviewer.**

SCENARIO 5

Prompt for Student

You are a primary care physician in a small town. One of your long-term patients comes to you and tells you that he wants to travel to India to undergo elective cosmetic surgery, because it is much cheaper to have the procedure done there than in the U.S. **Consider the pros and cons to this choice and how you would discuss them with the patient. Enter the room and discuss this with the interviewer.**

SCENARIO 6

Prompt for Student

You are entering a debate about whether CRNAs should be able to do everything that Anesthesiologists do. The Veterans Affairs Administration is considering removing physician Anesthesiologists from the operating room and replacing them with CRNAs. **Enter the room and discuss with the interviewer. You are to argue against this, and discuss why you don't think CRNAs should be given the same responsibilities as physician Anesthesiologists.**

SCENARIO 7

Prompt for Student

You are a physician working in the Emergency Department. Your 15-year-old patient has suffered severe blood loss from a deep laceration due to an ice skating accident; she is a Jehovah's Witness, and her mom has already told the hospital that she doesn't want her daughter to receive a blood transfusion. The patient needs a blood transfusion immediately if there is any hope of saving her life. **Enter the room and discuss with the interviewer what you would say to the mom to help her understand that her daughter needs the blood transfusion.**

CHAPTER 23

QUESTIONS TO ASK THE INTERVIEWER

At the end of most interviews, the interviewer will give you the opportunity to ask questions. This is your time to shine! Asking questions not only gives you more time to build rapport with the interviewer, but it allows you the opportunity to be memorable. Asking a question that continues the dialogue can be the difference between the interviewer remembering key details about you when she argues your case in front of the rest of the Admissions Committee, or forgetting about you.

The biggest mistake I see students make when it comes to asking the interviewer questions is asking very specific, very nuanced questions that the interviewer may not be able to answer. Sure, the interviewer can say that she will find out for you, but it's a conversation stopper. You have to understand that not everyone interviewing you will have an intimate knowledge of the curriculum changes, or the student-run clinic, or research going on at the school.

Asking more general, opinion based questions allows for anyone to answer them, and doesn't require specific knowledge.

- Do you believe the faculty and administration are happy with the current curriculum, or do you feel there are areas that they might want to change?
- Would you want your daughter or son to attend school here?
- What is one thing about this school that more people should know about?
- What special programs is this school known for?
- Do you believe that students have sufficient involvement in the school's major committees, such that their voices are heard and acted upon?
- What do you feel is the best part of the medical school?
- If I were to ask the graduating medical students, what would they say was the best part of being a student here?
- If I were to ask the graduating medical students, what would they say was the one thing that best prepared them for residency?
- Where do you see there being major changes at this school over the next four years?
- How does this school compare to your alma mater? (assuming the interviewer is a physician and didn't go to this school)
- If I were to poll the faculty, what would they say is the biggest area needing improvement at this school?
- Can I look at the Match list for the last couple of years?

CHAPTER 24

QUESTIONS TO ASK THE MEDICAL STUDENTS

Medical students attending the school you are interviewing at, are a gold mine of information. Remember that you typically will only spend a day at each campus, which isn't a lot of time to gather enough information to make the most informed decision. To better help you make that decision, why not go straight to the people who were in your shoes not that long ago?

One thing to keep in mind is that every encounter that you have with medical students (or anyone else on the campus) can get back to the Admissions Committee. Even though you are having a conversation with someone your age, in a more relaxed environment, keep it professional.

Here are some ideas of questions to ask the students.

- Where do students usually live during the first and second years?
- Do you need a car to get around?

- What note taking services do you have?
- Is class mandatory?
- What percentage of classes are mandatory?
- Are there small breakout sessions for problem-based learning?
- What do you like best about being a student here?
- What do you like least about being a student here?
- What do you wish you knew before coming here?
- If you had the choice between this school and [insert another school that is your top choice], which one would you choose?
- How soon after you started did you have interaction with patients?
- Are faculty members available outside of the classroom?
- How receptive are the faculty members to feedback?
- What is the cost of living in this area?
- Where do students go to relax?
- How much bonding is there among the students?
- If you could change one thing about the school, what would it be?
- How is the rotation selection for the third and fourth years?
- Did you get the electives and rotations that you wanted, in the order that you wanted?
- How far away are clinical rotations?
- Do you have to move or temporarily live somewhere else during clinical rotations?
- Do you have to find your own clinical rotations for main rotations, like surgery or internal medicine?
- How are the medical students treated during clinical rotations?
- Do you find that you have enough time to do everything?
- Is there a gym on campus?
- What airport do people fly in/out of?
- How long does it normally take to get to the airport?
- How is the on-campus housing? (assuming there is on-campus housing)
- How do you like the cafeteria food? (assuming there is a cafeteria on campus)
- Are the courses fixed, or can you pick what courses you want to take?

- Was a mentor assigned to you?
- Do you think that students who need extra time or other accommodations are treated fairly?
- Do you know of any students who have failed, and if so, how has the school accommodated them?
- How diverse do you think the student body is?
- How are you evaluated during your non-clinical years?
- How are you evaluated during your clinical years?
- Tell me about the library. Do many students study there?
- Where is the best place to study?
- Is parking an issue?
- Do you think that you are provided with good education when rotating in the hospital, or do you get more of a sense that you are in the way?
- How are the facilities in the hospital for call nights?
- Where do students go to decompress after tests?
- What is a normal lunch served on campus?
- Are you happy? Are most students happy here?
- How much time do you get to study for Step/Level 1?
- Did the school provide you with resources for Step/Level 1?
- What does fourth year look like?
- Where do students go for fun?

SECTION III

THE EXAMPLES

CHAPTER 25

TELL ME ABOUT YOURSELF

The biggest mistakes that I see students make in answering this question are: 1) sounding too rehearsed—which is what we talked about in an earlier part of this book, and 2) sounding like they're reading their application or their resume, going step-by-step through their application.

Let me give you an example. I recently did an interview with a student, which I started by saying, "So tell me about yourself." And his response was, "Well, I grew up in this town, then I went to college, and I did X, then Y, and finally Z. Then I went to this job, and I worked for this long. Then I started volunteering, and did this, and then I really wanted to pursue medicine so I went back and did my post-baccalaureate, and after that I did this and that."

That's not how you should be answering the "Tell me about yourself" question. They have your application. They have either read it before your interview, or they'll read it after. Answering with a chronological account of your life doesn't allow a conversation to start, which is what you want to happen. You want a conversation, and that won't be possible if you are regurgitating your application or your resume.

This is your opportunity to tell the interviewer something exciting about you. Show them what you've done, and share something memorable about you. I say "show," because the more stories that you can weave in, the better. Humans love and respond to stories. They are memorable, and you want to be memorable enough that your interviewer will want to advocate for you in front of the Admissions Committee. What's your favorite movie? What's your favorite sport? Where's the most interesting place you've ever been? Tell them something that they're going to remember you by, something that no one else is going to say. That's who you are. Are you a twin? Do you have great family stories? Use these anecdotes, whatever they may be. This is your opportunity to shine. Each of those unique aspects are little threads that you're leaving for the interviewer to pull on to go deeper into the conversation. This is exactly what you want!

STUDENT A

The following three answers are from the same student, over three different interviews. You'll be able to see how his answers improved each time. Read the feedback I gave him to get a sense of what I was thinking about his answer.

Interview 1

Ryan: Why don't you tell me a little bit about yourself?

Student A: I think the best place to start is my family. I have a really large family. There are eight of us total, four brothers and a sister. My dad and mom are from Argentina and Chile, respectively, and that's where I became who I am. I learned from them at a young age. Some of the things that I think best represent who I am, is I was able to go to school in Washington, and play soccer there, because I'm South American and that's what South Americans do.

One of the things that I really love doing is being involved in a teaching setting. I did a lot of mentoring and tutoring throughout college, and I just love to learn. I'm really passionate about learning about not just science and medicine, but I love philosophy and I love psychology. Those are some brief, some brief little tidbits about who I am, but I think they represent me fairly accurately.

Feedback

You talked about your family, which is great. I liked how you said, "That's where I became who I am." I liked your description about playing soccer up in Washington. Then you took this twist and told me about yourself, including some interesting details, but then you started to give me a resume trying to show me why you're qualified for medicine, which is a common mistake. You started talking about some of your extracurricular activities, about teaching and mentoring, and your love of learning. From the interviewer's standpoint, I take that as you're here to sell me on your application.

At this point in the game, you don't need to sell me on the application. You're obviously there for an interview. They like you enough to have you there. It's just a matter of communicating at that point some other things that aren't in your application, so details about your family are good. Soccer is definitely something that sets you apart, that you were a student athlete in college. What other cool things are there about you that you can add into that? Travel experiences, hobbies, anything else, and then tie it back to medicine. What are you doing in this seat today? Why am I interviewing you? So, you have a big family, you love to play soccer, you love teaching and mentoring, great. Where did medicine come about? Usually you can work in that medicine exposure somewhere in your tell me about yourself.

Interview 2

Ryan: Why don't you tell me a little bit about yourself, and what brought you here today?

Student A: I think the best place to start is with my family. That's essentially where I developed not only my skills, but also my character traits and who I am today. I come from a big family. There are eight of us total. I have four brothers and a sister. My parents are interesting, because they emigrated from Argentina and Chile, so there's a lot of culture behind the family I grew up in. It was a lot of fun, but it was also interesting growing up in the States while having that background.

Some of the things that I really enjoy doing: So, because I'm South American, soccer is the first thing that comes to mind. The thing that I've done ever since I could walk, basically. I had the opportunity to not only play soccer in high school but in college as well. I went to a school in Washington State, and I played there. I had a wonderful time and developed probably some of my strongest friendships in that area—because you're with them so much, you know. You literally bleed and sweat [laughter] with them. And rise to the challenge when need be.

One of the things that I enjoy doing is listening to people's stories, so one of the ways I can do that now is through listening to podcasts. It's a really strong way for me to connect with a lot of different cultures and a lot of different diverse backgrounds. It's also a way that I can continue to learn, everything from the Radiolab I just finished to a series called Serial, that was absolutely fascinating, and just a wonderful piece of journalism.

And the last thing that I would say that I really enjoy doing, and that represents me well, is that I like to build things. When I was young, we actually built our house in a traditional South American fashion. It's made with cinder blocks. Not wood, but cinder blocks. It's a 2,500-square foot home, two stories, entirely of cinder blocks. So you're looking at one foot by one foot blocks that you essentially have to lay on top of each other. And so from a young age, I was able to do that. It all comes back to family, because I think the reason that I really enjoy doing that is that I had the opportunity to do it with my father.

Back in 2008, my father got sick, and in 2012 he underwent aortic transplant surgery. Now I take every single chance that I get to go back and work with him, and be in an environment where I can be with him and work with my hands. I really value that. That's when I would say that my intrigue and my passion for medicine really all began—when my dad got sick.

Feedback

This was a very similar answer to your previous answer, the way you started out by talking about your family. Family is obviously the core of your being. That comes across very strongly. The answer here was good, but it was long. So now the question is, how do we cut out the excess—even though we know it's good—because shorter is better in this situation. You told a great story, and my notes specifically say, "Great story—long."

And then you got into your dad getting sick. So it went even longer, and I thought we were wrapping up. We'll have to shorten that. Go back and watch it and see. I don't know if the whole "stories" part is necessary, like loving stories, and so on.

But that's what got you talking about podcasts, which is intriguing and different, because then we started talking about Serial, which is obviously totally off the cuff. That's what you want to do during these interviews. Serial was one of the hottest things going last year. Everybody was talking about it. And so, if you get an interviewer who loved Serial too, then sure, go talk about Serial for half the interview. That's awesome. It was all good. It was just long.

Interview 3

Ryan: Tell me about yourself.

Student A: I think the important place to start is with my family. I come from a large family. There are eight people in my family—four brothers, three older and one younger, and a little sister. And one of the great things about my family is that my parents are South American. My dad is Chilean, and my mom is Argentine.

And for those reasons, two things are certain. Good food and soccer. So the one thing that I'm good at – because I can't cook – is playing soccer. And I did that luckily all through life and into college. And it gave me the opportunity to play soccer at the [redacted] University in [redacted]. That was a huge blessing. And it helped develop my character of who I am now. And that's where some of my best friendships actually came to be.

I think the second really important thing that defines me is my love for building. And this one's also pretty closely linked to my family as well. It's something that I learned from my dad. We built our house. It's handmade. We made it out of cinder block—it's concrete one foot by one foot blocks, twenty-five hundred square feet. Huge house, beautiful. And I helped him build that. And any chance that I get now to go back and help my dad build, whether it's a doghouse, as simple as that, or whether it's renovating an apartment that they own—I relish it.

Because in 2008, my dad was diagnosed with heart disease. In 2012, he had aortic bypass surgery. And that linked me even closer to my family. Something that's really representative of who I am, but it also ignited my love for medicine and pretty much steered me down that path.

Ryan: How's your dad doing now?

Student A: He's doing well. He's recovered really well from the surgery.

Feedback

Ryan: That's much, much better. Short, sweet, to the point, interesting. I liked it. One of the interesting things that you could add to this is the fact that you not only played soccer at [name of college redacted], but you also coached. When you were twenty-two or twenty-three, graduating college, that's when you were the coach?

Student A: Yes.

Ryan: You had to be the youngest coach."

Student A: There were players on the team who were older than me. Three of them, I think. Three players who were twenty-six. I was the youngest coach they ever hired in the history of the university.

Ryan: It's a huge spin for you. That shows you have supervisory skills, leadership skills, organizational skills. All that can be thrown in, by adding that to your "tell me about yourself."

STUDENT B

The following four answers are from the same student, over four different interviews. You'll be able to see how his answer improved each time. Read my feedback to him to get a sense of what I was thinking about his answer.

Interview 1

Ryan: Why don't we start by having you tell me a little bit about yourself?

Student B: Well, my name is [redacted]. I'm twenty-seven and I live here in Seattle with my spouse of five years, and my two dogs, a Shiba Inu and a Siberian husky. I'm very much a naturalist at heart. Some of my hobbies include hiking, camping, fishing, anything on the water pretty much. I'm also a scuba dive master. I help teach new scuba divers around the Puget Sound area here. I'm also a musician. I trained since I was four years old on the piano, and I really love to play classic rock. I grew up in Iowa, in a classic Midwest Catholic farming family. I'm the first in my family to go to a four-year university. I graduated in March with a degree in biology. I didn't go to college right after high school. I joined the military, where I served as a combat medic for five years.

My last duty station was in Tacoma, which is just south of Seattle, and after I got out I moved to Seattle and I've been here ever since.

Feedback

Ryan: You did a good job by not giving me a resume. You didn't go through your path of, "I did this and then I did this, and then I did this," but you did give me a lot of information. But when you began, you said your name is [redacted]. They know your name. You don't need to say your name, other than when you first shake hands and you introduce yourself. You talked about being married, having your dogs, being a naturalist, everything you do there, being a musician, graduating from college … You got into a little bit of a timeline-resume recounting at the end, when talking about graduating. Then you reversed it, by going back into your military career after high school, so just be careful about those timeline-type statements. I would pick some of the highlights and focus on those, so that you don't give a very long answer."

Interview 2

Ryan: Why don't you tell me a little bit about yourself?

Student B: I live in Seattle with my spouse of the past five years. We have two dogs, a Shiba Inu and a Siberian husky. I'm very much a naturalist. I love everything outdoors. I do a lot of hiking and backpacking, camping here in the Pacific Northwest. I'm also a scuba diver. I'm a petty dive master—I help train new scuba divers and teach them about environmental concerns, and how to lessen their impact under water. I'm also a cyclist. I do meditate to long-term cycle rides ... one hundred to two hundred miles or so. My most recent was a ride called RSVP, from Seattle to Vancouver, British Columbia. That was a rather fun ride over a really long hill, and into another country, which is an exciting way to do a ride. I'd never done that before.

I'm from Iowa. I come from a large Midwest, Catholic, farming family. After high school, I went to college for a semester, and I realized it wasn't for me. I joined the military, where I served as a combat medic. I really enjoyed my time in the military. I got to travel and see a lot of things. I learned a lot about myself, and about my passion for medicine. I got out in 2013, and I've been in Seattle ever since.

Feedback

When you go back and listen to this, listen to how you introduce your nature background, the way you talk about camping, the way you talk about diving. There's a lot of "and I also ... and I also ... and I also," which could be wrapped up succinctly by saying, "I love the outdoors. I love nature, pretty much anything about it. I love camping, and bike riding, and canoeing, and diving," and you could tie it all together, with a prettier bow, instead of how you've been doing it.

You also left out the reason that you're sitting here today, so I could have easily followed up that question again, as I did last time with, "Why medicine?" Okay, great to know that's who you are, but what are you doing here today? So you can tie that in; you can talk about your history and say "I was in the Army for X number of years and had a lot of exposure to medicine; at some point I knew that being a physician was my calling, what I really wanted to do. So, I got out of the military and rededicated myself to my premedical studies, and that's why I'm here." Something along those lines.

Interview 3

Ryan: Tell me about yourself.

Student B: Well, I've lived in Seattle with my spouse for the past five years. We have two dogs, a Shiba Inu and a Siberian husky. I am definitely a naturalist at heart. I love doing everything outside, hiking, camping, scuba diving, cycling, pretty much anything I can do outside. Living here in the Pacific Northwest has really allowed me to explore that unhindered, and I'm really thankful that I've been here for that.

I also really like music. I play the piano. I particularly like to play classic rock, Eric Clapton, Billy Joel, Elton John, that kind of music. I don't like to pursue my love of nature out in the rain, so music is my peace of mind and my go-to activity when I don't want to go outside in the rain.

It hasn't always been like that. I grew up in Iowa in a small farming community. My family's Catholic, and I have a lot of brothers and sisters. I left Iowa when I joined the military. I spent a lot of time – five years – in the military. I was a combat medic and I really, really enjoyed my experience. It helped me to mature, to grow up, to learn a lot about myself, and it helped me explore medicine. I learned a lot about the medical field and my role in it.

I got a lot of patient care experience, a lot of one-on-one, and I worked with other physicians, both allopathic and osteopathic physicians. And that time really helped me develop my excitement around joining the medical field, and that's ultimately what led me to finish school when I got out of the military. And that led me here today to the interview to go to medical school at [redacted].

Feedback

Ryan: I'm still feeling that this is a little disjointed. (In the feedback to this question we jumped around a lot, which is why I didn't put anything succinct in the feedback for this response. The gist of the feedback was that it was still a little all over the place, and it needed to be summed up a little better.)

Interview 4

Student B: Well, I live here in Seattle with my partner of the past six years and my two dogs, a Shiba Inu and a Siberian husky. I'm very much a naturalist at heart. I love doing everything outside, from hiking to camping, boating, scuba diving, cycling – you name it.

Ironically, living here in Seattle, I don't really like being out in the rain, but that allows me to explore another passion I have – music. I've played the piano since I was four. Ah, I love playing classic rock, Elton John, Billy Joel, Eric Clapton kind of music.

I come from Iowa. I'm from a large Catholic Iowa farming family. I did a lot of this outdoor stuff when I was child, and that's probably what spawned my enthusiasm for it as an adult. I was in the Boy Scouts and became an Eagle Scout.

When I was nineteen, I joined the military. I served for five years as a combat medic and I thoroughly enjoyed that experience. It allowed me to explore and discover my passion for medicine in a unique way that a lot of people don't have the opportunity to do, because in the military you get these unique opportunities for patient interactions and patient care.

That was a great opportunity for me, and that really set forth my plans for the future. When I got out of the military, I finished my undergraduate degree, and that's what led me here today, to interviewing for medical school.

Feedback

Ryan: Much better! Short and to the point. You hit all the highlights that you wanted. You talked about the military and your exposure to medicine which is what brought you here today, so that's good.

STUDENT C

The following four answers are from the same student, over four different interviews. You'll be able to see how her answer improved each time. Read my feedback to the applicant to get a sense of what I was thinking about her answers.

Interview 1

Ryan: Why don't you start off by telling me a little bit about yourself?

Student C: I think my sister captures my personality really well when she calls me a Renaissance woman. I have an appreciation for a variety of arts. I'm very athletic, and I also love listening to people's stories. I've always been a very humanistic person, and compassionate and creative. When I call myself an artist – from a young age I always enjoyed painting and then throughout my years in elementary school and again intermittently in college, I've continued with it. And it really reflects my ability to see issues from different perspectives. I feel like when I'm painting, I'm in this zone where I can just be alone with the canvas, but really zoom in on this image.

And then in my athletics, I've been an athlete my whole entire life. I grew up as a tennis player traveling the California coast playing competitive tournaments. And it's really cultivated this determination and focus in me, and I have this ability to fight through challenges. And I think a pivotal moment in my career was being able to play at the collegiate level and making a really big impact on my team as a team member, and also serving as a leader. So again, I love athletics. Since college I've turned into a runner and have competed in various distances. I just love the physical and mental challenge of athletics, and that's something that I will pursue my whole life.

Again, I've said I'm a creative person. I love coming home at the end of the day and trying out new recipes in the kitchen. I grew up in the kitchen with my mother and grandmother, helping them cook. I've since learned a lot and developed a real fascination with health and nutrition. And that's led me to this pathway today, because I did not take sciences in college and I did not foresee myself becoming a doctor until a lot more recently. Then again, I'm a really humanistic person, I love interacting with people and hearing people's stories.

I volunteer with the homeless in free park clinics on a weekly basis, and I feel like I can bring a lot to the table, just being able to listen to their stories and struggles, and just being there to hear their stories. So that's a little bit about me in a nutshell.

Feedback

Ryan: "Tell me about yourself," – it's the hardest question to start with, right? Talking about yourself. That's where I felt that this agenda that you had came out.

I like how you started out by talking about being a Renaissance woman, being artistic and athletic, and listening to people's stories. And then it turned into you trying to highlight yourself. So you're selling yourself to the interviewer. You talked about how you have this ability to see things from different perspectives.

Talking about your ability, you started talking about your tennis career and how that's taught you to fight through challenges and serve as a leader. You're selling yourself to the interviewer, instead of just telling a story. Tell a story about yourself.

It was very long, because you had an agenda of, "I need to tell him this, and I need to tell him this, and I need to tell him that." But the "Tell me about yourself " question is your opportunity to communicate how you are different.

This is your time to shine. You're a nontraditional student. You have a lot to prove, to show that you're different from all the other applicants coming through. Your artistic and athletic background make you unique. You can talk about playing tennis. You can talk about loving to run and loving to cook. You've got lots to say. Talk about fun hobbies, fun travel experiences, talk about your family, your sisters, anything that's different about you. Mention that you're from the area—obviously it's a huge tie for [redacted].

That's where we need to focus on your "Tell me about yourself" question – a lot less selling of yourself and a lot more offering a story about how you're different.

Take some highlights about how you're different and craft that. Being an athlete and a competitive tennis player is interesting and unique. I have my knowledge of tennis, and I love watching the Grand Slam events. I was thinking, "Okay, I know some tennis. Let's talk tennis." That's exactly where you want your "Tell me about yourself" to lead your interviewer—to a personal connection, into an easy, flowing conversation. "That's super, you play tennis? I play tennis too. I hurt my shoulder, I blew out my knee," and that kind of thing. Before you know it, the time is up, and you just had a conversation with an old buddy for half an hour.

Student C: Should I shorten my "Tell me about yourself," and just touch on less information and go into more depth? Or is it better to have more things, less in-depth? What's best?

Ryan: Shorter. Highlights. What is different and unique about you? What might you want to continue talking about?

Interview 2

Ryan: Why don't you tell me a little bit about yourself?

Student C: First of all, I just want to say I'm very excited to be here. It's a pleasure to meet you. I grew up in Southern California, the middle of three sisters. I'm very close with my family. My sisters and I have a very tight bond, and I remember the time my sister called me a Renaissance woman. She regards me as someone with a diverse range of interests. I'm an artist, an athlete and I'm also really curious about exploring new areas. I've never ... I've never shied away from new opportunities.

I grew up loving to paint. I painted throughout elementary school. In high school I took art; then in college during vacations I'd come home and train with a local artist, and I've learned a lot through my exploration. My art allows me to express myself in a visual format which is really pleasing for me. And then also I've always loved to sing. In elementary school I had an incredibly inspirational music teacher, and that followed me through high school. I participated in three different choral groups, and in my last semester of college I was able to participate in an a capella group.

I feel like I really excelled with the camaraderie of working towards a common goal with a group of people who share my joy of singing. I've also been a pianist. I played piano throughout college as well, and I think my athletic career as a tennis player really defines in me too, as I grew up and learned important lessons through playing women's tennis at a competitive level. I trained pretty much the last fifteen years to play at the competitive collegiate level, and I eventually succeeded in fulfilling that goal, so I've had some proud moments there.

Growing up, in the summers sometimes I trained six hours a day on the court, as well as every day after school during the school year. I traveled around the California coast on weekends playing tournaments, looking for challenging competition and again, it was a huge part of my college experience. Athletics has always been a big part of my life. And then since college, I've turned to running and I've found a lot of solace and also time to think. Just going out on the road alone sometimes and getting in those endorphins [laughter]."

Ryan: That's good.

Student C: I also have always had a passion for stories and listening to people tell me about their history, and I think that comes into play a lot when I work. Right now I'm volunteering in the park clinics, after work one night a week, and I just love it. I love being with a diverse group of people, including the volunteers who help and listen to their stories and are just there for them. That's made a huge impact on my life and my career path. So that's a little bit about me in a nutshell.

Feedback

Ryan: Your "tell me about yourself" is still very long.

Student C: Yes, I felt that. I was like, wait, do I say one more thing?

Ryan: Yes, and I interrupted. I was wondering, "Oh, is she done yet? Nope, still going." So we need to figure out how to pare it down. A lot of your stories about singing and being a pianist and painting can be dialed down into one or two sentences, just about your artistic expression. You start off by talking about being a Renaissance woman—the artist in you. You love expressing yourself musically by playing the piano and singing, you love expressing yourself by painting, and so on. You don't need to draw it out. At one point you started talking about how you took painting classes in high school and college. I don't need to know that. That doesn't give me a good story about you. Just highlight that.

That's where a lot of the length of your "tell me about yourself" answer came in. When you talk about tennis, remember you want this to be as conversational as possible. So you want to throw out these little threads of, "Oh I love to paint, and I love to sing, and I love to do all these things … I'm a competitive tennis player." Let them pull on those threads and get more out of you instead of you going on for too long. You talked about training six hours a day in the summer and traveling on the weekends, and it just went on and on and on about tennis.

Just talk about being a competitive tennis player and the experiences that that has afforded you. Just give a very brief synopsis about the teamwork involved or whatever you want to highlight. The fact that you won that match last year, that it was down to you—that's a good little story. What highlights, what accolades have you received as a tennis player? Can you say, "I was a collegiate champion tennis player?" Give that highlight, and then let them ask the questions and make it a conversation.

Student C: So I should say I was a tennis player and even got to pursue it in college? And then say a pivotal moment in my career was this match? And should I talk about the championship match?

Ryan: You could tell a nice little tidy story all around that. Yes. And you weren't just a tennis player, you were a competitive women's tennis player. And did you get a scholarship for that?

Student C: No. There were no scholarships, so unfortunately not.

Ryan: Okay. Were you recruited to [redacted] to play tennis?

Student C: Yes.

Ryan: Then you could talk about that. Not a lot of students applying to medical school are athletes who have been recruited to college. So you can talk about how you were ... how you were lucky enough to get recruited to go play in college and tell the story of your athletics there."

Interview 3

Ryan: Why don't you tell me a little bit about yourself?

Student C: I was born and raised in Southern California. I am the middle of three girls and I'm very close with my family. My family describes me as a Renaissance woman. I love to express myself through painting and art. I've also played the piano, and I sang in the choir throughout my educational career in high school and college. I made a lot of close friends in choir, and I think one of the reasons I really enjoyed it was the teamwork aspect and collaboration with other individuals towards a common goal. I think that was also part of my motivation throughout childhood to pursue collegiate tennis, being able to contribute to a team environment in something that I love to do. In college I did have the opportunity at [redacted]—I was recruited to play on the tennis team, and I learned so many life lessons both on and off the court. But one of the pivotal moments in my collegiate career was winning the championship tournament at the [redacted]. For me and my team, I was the last match on court, all eyes were on me, and I was the underdog that pulled it out. That's a memory I really treasure, that was a really great moment for me and my team.

Since college I've turned to running. I loved competing and distance events. It gives me time to meditate on my own, but I've also been fortunate to have a broad array of clinical experiences. I worked at Planned Parenthood, with diverse populations, and I volunteered with Doctors Without Walls, and participated as a member on the street medicine team. That has been a phenomenal experience, seeing so many different people and their struggles and talking to them and, and learning their backgrounds and why they are there and how we can help in our communities.

In my free time I love to cook. I look forward to coming home at the end of the day and exchanging my scrubs for an apron and trying out new recipes. On weekends I like to garden and I planted some herbs. I have a broad range of interests. That's a little bit about me.

Feedback

Ryan: Probably your best one yet. You talked about where you were raised, a little bit about your family, the Renaissance part. The twist that you took when you mentioned the correlation with choir and teamwork and collaboration felt a little forced. Again, you fell back into your "I have these bullet points that I'm trying to convey," and so it felt a little forced. Then you brought it back to tennis. I like what you said about tennis. I like the championship discussion there. Then you talking about running, and you immediately jumped into having a broad array of clinical experiences and that felt very strange. Why did you go from running, to clinical experiences, and then back to cooking? It was very strange.

I think you can cut down a little bit. I don't think you need to mention gardening and cooking. Everything you said at the beginning was great, and after you bring it back to tennis you can go into your initial aspirations for a career involving nutrition. You can say, "When I was doing research for that, then exploring that, I actually met an osteopathic physician and was able to shadow her and see her interactions with patients and X, Y, and Z. And that's why I'm here."

Interview 4

Ryan: Why don't you tell me a little bit about yourself?

Student C: Well, I'm the middle of three girls, born and raised in California, and I'm very close with my family. My family always described me as a Renaissance woman because of my diverse interests. I love to express myself through painting, art, and music. I played the piano and sang in a number of choirs throughout my education. I'm also an athlete. I love the mental and physical challenge of competitive athletics, and I trained throughout my childhood as a competitive tennis player, and was fortunate to have the opportunity to be recruited at [redacted] College, where I played on the team and I learned a lot about myself, but I also discovered my potential as an athlete, which was really exciting and gratifying along with the team experience.

Some of my pivotal moments were on the tennis team breaking through tough matches and learning how to play under pressure, specifically my senior year at the [redacted] tournament when I was the last match on court. All eyes were on me, and I came back as the underdog and won the tournament for my team. So I have some good memories there. In college I worked really hard academically and actually majored in urban studies, not taking any sciences. It wasn't until well into my junior year that I had an internship opportunity and realized my desire to pursue medicine. And after college, I pursued post-baccalaureate courses in Santa Barbara in order to fill the prerequisites for medical school. During that time, I participated in a number of clinical experiences.

I worked at Planned Parenthood and counseled and educated young women making really tough decisions, and I volunteer currently for Doctors Without Walls, and I'm a member of the Street Medicine Team, which has been a really gratifying experience. I've seen people struggle and heard stories that have further inspired me to want to pursue medicine as my career. I work full-time as a medical assistant for a derm surgeon's office, where daily I'm having great patient contact, and counseling patients about their pathology reports. I'm also a runner, and I compete in distance events. And I look forward to the end of the day, when I have a little bit of time to be creative and come home and cook and explore in the kitchen. And that's a little bit about me.

Feedback

Ryan: I thought you did a good job here, up until a certain point. You started out great, talking about being a Renaissance woman, painting, art, music, piano, tennis. You said, 'I worked hard academically in college, actually an urban studies major,' so you were making that transition into where medicine came into play. And you talked about your internship. And then you started reciting your resume, right? "I'd worked at Planned Parenthood. I work in a street clinic. I work full time as an MA." Then you started ticking off things from your resume, and then you went back again into your athletics and your cooking.

So there was something in your head where you were thinking, "Oh, darn it. I forgot to mention running. And I forgot to mention cooking." And so you added that at the end and finished that way. But when you mention that you're a Renaissance woman and you love painting, art, and music, you mentioned the creativity of cooking – ultimately all of those things are creative expressions, right?

So, you can tie that in just at the beginning. "My family describes me as a Renaissance woman. I have a lot of creativity that I love to explore through cooking, painting, and music," and so on. And take care of it that way. Talk about your amazing tennis experience because that's a big part of who you are, and then switch to medicine, and end strong with medicine.

Student C: Okay, so you liked that I talked about the Planned Parenthood and the volunteering but just not the way I talked about it, or not at all?

Ryan: Those don't belong there. That's in your application. Those are experiences that are listed there. You don't need to bring them up in this situation. You talk about your exposure to the internship and the physician in the internship which is what you got you interested in medicine, how you went back and did your post-baccalaureate, and ultimately again, that's why you're here today. But all of the clinical experience and the things that you just mentioned don't belong there.

Student C: Okay. So I should still say that after college I did a post-baccalaureate and had a range of clinical opportunities that encouraged me to pursue medicine, but I don't have to say specifically what they were.

Ryan: Correct, you don't have to specifically say what they were.

Student C: Then maybe they'll probe further.

Ryan: They'll probe. Exactly! So that's where you want to leave these tiny little threads that they'll pull. "Tell me about those clinical experiences." "Tell me about XYZ."

CHAPTER 26

ANY RED FLAGS?

The dreaded red flags question! Do you air out all of your dirty laundry? Do you try to hide the worst of the worst? Do you try to give a little bit and hope that the interviewer doesn't ask any deeper questions? These are common questions that I get from students wondering how deep they should go.

Red flag questions are more common in closed interviews because the interviewer doesn't have access to your grades and your MCAT score before the interview. The closed interview typically has access to your essays and nothing more. They will have access to your full application after the interview, so don't think that you can hide something and they'll never know.

Let's assume you had to take the MCAT three times because you scored poorly the first two times and your third score still wasn't great (although you hope it's good enough).

How do you talk about this? Remember that you are at the interview, so the school has already screened your application and thinks that you have the ability to be part of next year's class. So maybe you think your MCAT score isn't good enough, but the school obviously does.

Instead of saying you have a low MCAT score, say your MCAT is below the school's average. While you are saying the same thing in the end, the latter sounds less negative.

What you don't want to do, with any red flags that you talk about, is talk about your bad grades, your below-average MCAT, any disciplinary action, etc., and not offer any sort of personal growth that you were able to achieve from the misstep.

Always talk about what you learned from your mistakes or struggles. The interviewer wants reassurance that you won't make the same mistake twice.

Another huge mistake that students make is not taking personal responsibility when talking about poor grades, dropped classes, or other troubles on their transcript.

Blaming the professor for your poor grade is not something that will win over your interviewer. I don't care if the class average was fourteen percent and the professor was fired at the end of the semester. You were responsible for your grade. You were responsible for not studying properly for the test that was given. Please don't blame or point fingers in your interview.

Negativity is major red flag for interviewers and Admissions Committees. Don't self-deprecate, don't whine and don't complain!

STUDENT A

Student A: I can only think of a couple. I do have a relatively low MCAT score. I did only take it once, so there's that. I scored a 496 on the new MCAT, which is acceptable obviously, as I am here today and I think I showed some strengths in some areas. I also have a withdrawal in a Calculus 2 course at the University of [redacted], one summer. I withdrew from the course because it wasn't a requirement. That was my first opportunity to take summer courses, and I didn't really understand the workload and requirements of the summer course. It's much faster and higher paced. At that time, I was taking two other courses that both involved labs, and in order to succeed much more strongly in those classes, I decided to not take Calculus 2. I did very well on those other two courses, so I think it was a good move on my part."

Feedback

Ryan: The MCAT score, I don't know if it's a red flag. You even mentioned it while you were talking about it, you said "It was obviously good enough for me to get here" and I think that's how you have to look at it. I don't know if I'd call it a red flag.

So, instead of saying "a relatively low MCAT score," you can say that it's maybe a little bit lower than their average. It's pretty much saying the same thing, but in a little bit of a brighter light. Saying that you scored below average is better than saying you have a low score. I like how you said you had some strengths in some areas on the test. Your answer for calculus, and having the withdrawal in calculus – I wouldn't even bring that up as a red flag.

I think having a withdrawal is fine, and I didn't like your answer because medical school is fast and high paced, and the work load is demanding. You're telling me, the interviewer, that you struggled in calculus because it was too fast, high-paced, and demanding, and that's what medical school is going to be like. So now I'm questioning your ability to handle medical school. So stick with the MCAT. I wouldn't mention the calculus withdrawal. There are a thousand and one reasons to withdraw from a course.

Student A: Would it be okay that I scored lower than the average and that I definitely struggled with it, in preparing and taking the test? Would it be okay to mention that, or just stay clear of that struggle?

Ryan: It's all about spinning what you want to say, right? So it's whether or not you struggled with the test, versus you underestimated the amount of time it was going to take to study, or you underestimated the amount of content, or underestimated something else. So there's struggle versus underestimate, and which one of those sounds better?

Student A: Yeah. Underestimate, yeah.

Ryan: Yes, so just word it better. Obviously you can talk about how it's the new MCAT, right? You underestimated the volume of new material that the new

MCAT was going to use, and there was a lot of uncertainty because it was the new MCAT—with what the questions were going to look like and so on.

STUDENT B

Student B: The one that comes to mind is I that applied last application cycle, and my MCAT score wasn't as strong as other applicants, and I also applied late in the cycle. I think any Admissions Committee would look at that and probably think that someone, the individual who's applying, perhaps hadn't done their research or was naïve to the process, and that might be a red flag. When I applied, I knew that it was late and I knew my MCAT score maybe wasn't as competitive as other people's, but I just wanted to get a feel for what the application cycle was going to be like. So I wouldn't want that to be perceived as naiveté. But yeah, that might be a red flag.

Ryan: Minus the red flag as, as you stated, and the MCAT, does your application have any weaknesses?

Student B: That's a great question. I would say that I have good grades, solid grades. I also am aware of the areas where they could have been better. One of those areas was organic chemistry, where I got a C plus. I went to a quarter school, so for three quarters, equivalent to two semesters, that might be perceived as a weakness, however, personally I know how much that helped me in my academic process. I learned so much from that class. Going through the struggle of always trying to improve and not necessarily seeing it manifest itself in a grade, I grew a lot, and while maybe I didn't get the grade that I hoped to get, I wouldn't change that experience for anything.

Feedback

Ryan: This is always a hard question. How much do you call yourself out? How much do you say? Because perhaps they don't care about you applying late, they might not care about X, Y, and Z, so it's a hard question. I liked how you talked about applying last cycle, your MCAT not being as strong as perhaps it could be or should be. However, you said something like, "I knew I applied late, but I wanted to get a feel for what it was like." To the interviewer, that might make it sound like you're just there wasting their time. Do you know what I mean? The interview might be thinking, "I had to review one more application just because you wanted to see what it was like."

So, you can twist it around instead, and if you want to convey your meaning in a better way, you can say, "A red flag might be that I'm actually a reapplicant. I applied last year, although I happened to apply late." Was there a reason that you applied late?

Student B: Yeah, I was coaching the university soccer team.

Ryan: So you might say, "Yeah, I happen to be a reapplicant. One of my downfalls last year was that I applied late in the application cycle because I was asked to coach my college team as a first-year graduate. It was highly unusual, but it was something that they needed me to do, and so I did it. I still wanted to apply anyway, even though I knew I was late, because being a physician is what I want to do, and if there was even a small chance that I would get accepted, it was worth it."

So, with those good twists it's much better than saying something that will sound to them like, "I just wanted to waste your time."

"Are there any weaknesses in your application?" is somewhat similar to the red flags question. I like how you talked about having solid grades … but there's this organic chemistry grade. I liked how you gave it that spin and said, "I got the C plus, but you know what? I learned a lot from it." You talked about how much it helped you in your academic progress. You could have taken it one step further. Instead of saying that it helped you, what did it help you do? Did it help you learn how to prioritize better? Did it help you learn how to study more efficiently? You could have taken it that one step further and given me an example. Generally, during these interviews, whenever you're asked a question, if you can give an example with your answer, it just drives home your answer that much more. As human beings, we love stories, so if you can answer your question with a story, I'll remember that a lot more than someone else who just gives me a yes or no answer.

STUDENT C

Student C: Yes, I do have a red flag in my application, and I write about that in the application itself. So you're going to see an explanation but I don't mind sharing it now. When I first started school, I was young, like everybody else. I moved out when I was seventeen and got my own place. It was pretty much expected and I had a hard time with it, that first year. I wanted to go to college, I mean, I was dead-set on that, so I did. I already had a young family. Obviously young, because I was only eighteen when I started school.

I didn't do well. I failed, actually. I had a 1.0 GPA in the first semester, and I was academically dismissed the second semester. I was off for three years, I believe. I reapplied for admission, and I went back. Once again, it was three years later. My financial circumstances were still difficult—I was working a lot of hours, and I didn't put the priority on school that I needed to. I mean, quite honestly, I did much better after I went back. I didn't get any D's or F's, but I didn't do stellar either.

So you'd see over the course of my associate's degree, I ended with a 2.6 average, and that was the end of that. It ended with a very rough time in my life. My wife at the time, now my ex-wife, was having some advancing mental illnesses that made it difficult to continue, and honestly I thought that was the end of my scholastic career at that point. But twelve years later, I went back, and that's a mark of pride for me. So since I've gone back, I've held a 4.0 over eighty credit-hours with many full-time semesters, and I made the dean's list multiple times.

Feedback

Ryan: So you did a good job here by talking about lessons learned, right? Because then you flipped it and you basically said, "You know, moving forward, 12 years later, now I have a 4.0 GPA." You obviously figured something out in between the beginning and the end. So you did a good job there. I think you did a good job explaining what's in your file. Red flags in the file are very easy questions for blind interviewers to ask. So be very ready for that, and you were ready. I liked your answer!

STUDENT D

Student D: I guess the biggest red flag that I had was when I got a C in organic chemistry for the first time. And, just to clarify, I retook the class later, and I was an able to get an A, but when I got the C in my organic chemistry class, that was partly because of my health. I was always tired for some reason, and I'm assuming that was because of a high-sugar diet, and not doing any physical activities.

But the more significant reason was that I didn't have the discipline or scheduling ability at that time, and it took me a while in college during my third year to really find myself, to really establish what works best for me in terms of studying. And organic chemistry wasn't an easy class when I took it the first time. For me, when it really clicked was making flashcards in a program called ANKI.

Besides that, also going over the class notes before going to class, reviewing it afterwards, developing a strict schedule, and overall making it a habit, so that every day, when I get out of class, I go home, I check my work right away... It became a routine for me, and I filled out my GPA. In addition to having good health, my GPA improved because I developed a stricter study schedule, and I hope that when I get to medical school, that ability to study, that ability to have good study habits, will maintain."

Feedback

Ryan: So, you jumped right on it, you said you got a C in organic chemistry. Obviously for a DO school, you retook it, and you got an A-. So it doesn't really matter that you got a C in organic chemistry. Does it even matter that you mention it? It's in your transcript, so they're going to see it, but it's not calculated into your GPA.

Student D: It's not calculated, but you asked me for a red flag, and that was the only thing I could think of.

Ryan: There was one thing that I liked. Whenever you're asked, "What are your weaknesses? What are your red flags? What do you struggle with?" with any sort of negative spin that they're trying to push on you, you need to be able to own the issue, say, "Yep, I got a C in organic chemistry." You owned the problem.

You talked about what you did to fix the problem, and then you talked about what you will continue to do moving forward, what you've learned from it, and how you're going to apply that moving forward.

Because, as the interviewer, as the Admissions Committee member, I want to make sure that you're going to be a good student, obviously.

You did a good job. You talked about how you've learned, you've worked through your studying skills, and you were able to succeed.

CHAPTER 27

WHY MEDICINE?

You might think that answering this question will be easy. After all, you've just spent many years preparing yourself to get to this point. Unfortunately, most students approach this question with the wrong ideas. It's very easy for students to get mixed up about what they're saying and have interviewers ask more probing questions which might lead the student to the wrong conclusion.

In the examples below you'll see that I tried to corner the students when they gave me an answer that I felt was incomplete. You'll read in my feedback to the students more about how to properly formulate their responses so that there are no doubts in the interviewer's mind that you're certain you want to become a physician.

"I want to help people" is not an acceptable answer. You can help people by bagging groceries at the grocery store. You can help people by pumping gas. You can help people by giving them home loans at the bank. Helping people is only a part of the answer; it is not the full answer. "I love science" is not the only answer either. To make it this far and to have an interview obviously shows that you've liked science enough to get good-enough grades to get to this point. You don't have to love science to be a physician, you just have to be good at science.

The best answers to "Why Medicine?" always come down to the experiences that you have had with patients. You need to talk about how the interactions made you feel, how you were able to make a patient feel, and how you want to re-experience that every day of your life.

I've seen some discussion on whether or not "Why Medicine?" is different than "Why do you want to be a doctor?" I take these to be the same question. You are applying to medical school to be a physician. You're not applying to PA school; you're not applying to nursing school. To you, medicine means being a physician. Answer the question in that way.

Don't allow yourself to be probed with deeper questions like, "Why not be a PA?" or "Why not be a nurse?" You leave yourself open to these questions if you answer the question more generally about your interest in healthcare, rather than your interest in being a physician.

One thing you certainly don't want to do with this question is answer it with any sort of expectation of being in charge, or being the boss, or with any financial undertones.

Just because you're the physician doesn't mean you're the boss; it just means that you have the final say in the care of the patient. Just because you're a physician doesn't mean you're going to be rich; physicians are very well compensated, but if you look at satisfaction ratings, physicians are still very dissatisfied with their pay. If you're going into this career for financial reasons, stop reading this book now and find something else to do.

STUDENT A

Student A: So I think it's always been in the back of my mind, but after graduating and going through the rigorous biomedical engineering curriculum, I wanted to get a job, and figure out what it's like to work as an engineer in the actual work force. So I started doing that and I realized it wasn't all that it was cracked up to be. I didn't have that dedication, the passion that I knew I wanted to have in my career, that one I'd be working forty-plus hours a week on.

So I knew there was something more out there, and I had to try becoming a doctor because I definitely think it would be a wonderful fit for me, and as I continued to volunteer, I wholeheartedly understood that I was going to do whatever it took to become a doctor."

Feedback

Ryan: You talked about that being always in the back of your mind, and you wanted to enter the workforce. Those are all solid answers because they're true. I would be leery of saying that you didn't have the dedication and passion for engineering because it'll lead to that question of, "Well, what's going to prevent you from losing dedication and passion for medicine, and are you just going to try this and decide you don't want to do it?"

It's a very common trap. You have to watch out for the verbiage that you're using, if it's the negative side of things.

You need to come from the positive side, like this: "Even though I've liked my job and have done well and enjoyed working as part of a team and doing all these great projects, there was something that continued to bug me about medicine, and these are the things that ultimately drove me to make that decision to switch."

STUDENT B

Student B: After my junior year of college, I realized ... I was an urban studies major first of all, a multi-disciplinary major focusing in art history and geography, so I was studying people in relation to their environment and place, thinking I was going to go into architecture.

But I became disillusioned with architecture and started thinking, "Well, what do I want to pursue? What do I love to read about? What do I love to learn about? What makes me tick?" And I realized I'm really fascinated by nutrition. I grew up watching my mom and grandma cook in the kitchen. I've always loved food, I love talking about food and creating new recipes at home, and I am especially interested in the link between being an athlete and food and how what we eat can affect our performance. And so I decided I wanted to see where I could go with that, and I found an internship opportunity in town at the Samsung Diabetes Research Institute. They have a nutritionist who works with their diabetic patients, so I applied for that.

They welcomed me for an internship and they said, "You know what? We have a premedical internship that you could join as well." I got to shadow local physicians through that, and I got to do research with one of the leading experts in diabetes research. I even got to help her with a publication, which was really a great experience. The most poignant moment though was accompanying her to the county clinic where she saw women with gestational diabetes. That really struck me as something special because these women were coming from a range of socioeconomic backgrounds, and most of them didn't even speak fluent English. But she really met them at eye level.

She sat with them, held their hands, and went through their journal entries where they mapped out their meal plans and went through everything and said, "Okay, I think we could substitute ingredients here, change a couple of things here." She took a really holistic perspective on her patients and that really impressed me. It struck me at that moment that that's what I wanted to do. I wanted to teach people about how they could lead healthier lives. This physician was a DO, so that's also when I first learned about osteopathic medicine. She mentored me at the beginning stages of my interest in this career path.

Ryan: Interesting. What you were describing about mentoring patients and educating patients—you could do that as a nutritionist. Why not be a nutritionist? What is your interest in taking all of those extra steps to become a physician?

Student B: I guess I forgot to mention it, but during the course of the internship I did get to do some research and learn more about the science of medicine. I became really fascinated with the idea of not only treating patients at a clinical level but also doing medical research and seeing how we can come up with new technologies, new devices and ways of helping people. I feel like being a physician really facilitates that, and I'll have the knowledge and skills to be able to pursue both paths. I did think briefly about being a nutritionist and then I thought, you know what? I think that's a little too easy. I want to do something more than just counsel nutrition. Then I realized I'm really fascinated with science at a deeper level, and I want to pursue being a physician.

Feedback

Ryan: The way you answered at first made me think, "You could be a nutritionist and do that."

What is it about medicine? And then, even your follow-up answer to that was about doing the research, which you can do as a nutritionist. There was something else there, and then you answered it. You said being a nutritionist is a little too easy. And that's more of a negative statement, right? That's putting down the nutritionists.

You can spin it and say that you were able to gain experience shadowing nutritionists, and you were able to see how they work, and you were able to gain the experience shadowing the osteopath.

Student B: It's more fulfilling.

Ryan: More fulfilling for you personally? Make it about you. Don't put down the nutritionists. So it's more fulfilling for you, it's more mentally stimulating for you. You feel you could have a bigger impact on your patients being able to not only counsel them on nutrition but also with all of their other health-related issues, as their physician. So just take it up to that next level.

STUDENT C

Interview 1

Student C: I guess my path to medicine started when I did my hospital internship, and the hospital internship allowed me to explore various departments from med-surg to ER to pediatrics. What really got me into it was the patient interaction I had when I first got there. The internship told me that I'd be exposed to a lot of things, see some cool things, maybe, but what really got me interested was just talking to patients, because, more often than not, there were a lot of times where I'd have no assignments going on, so I would just walk around and talk to patients, making sure everything was okay. It was just the chance to listen to their stories, and see why they're there, and trying to make sure that everything is okay for them, trying to make sure that they're comfortable, and just helping them recover.

It was very rewarding to be part of a team, and from that experience, I knew that being a healthcare professional, pursuing something in health, was something that I wanted to do, and working on the medical scribe later on, I learned more about the roles and responsibilities of a doctor. I followed them around, did live charting and worked in the EMR, and I realized that it was very stressful to become a doctor, with the amount of work they have to do. I feel that, besides helping other people, I like the aspect of using your science background, using my knowledge to diagnose or figure out the problem—that's also very appealing to me.

Finally, what really made me choose osteopathic medicine was the shadowing. In the hospital, I wasn't able to really distinguish between these different kinds of healthcare professionals. They were practically identical in what they did. So, shadowing allowed me to explore more of the OMT in particular, and it also allowed me to discuss with a doctor about the holistic approach, the idea of philosophy. Some of them talked about their belief in the whole body unity, and their belief that something could have really prevented needing to take medicine, and I really took that to heart. It was a combination of all these events that led me to where I am today, and I really want to put it out there because of that.

Ryan: I'm interested. Your first comment was that it was the hospital internship that drove you into medicine, but something had to be there to drive you to do the hospital internship. There had to be something else that was driving you towards health care…

Student C: Well, as a biology major, you encounter plenty of students who are premed, pre-pharm, and so on, and they always ask you, "So, what do you want to do, later on?" And I was exposed to the whole, "after science, do health, later on in life," but, a particular event in my Circle K club – a community service club at my school – was important to me. We did a bone marrow drive, and through that event I was able to interact with one of the doctors there. It was a very simple conversation, but I was very surprised that, even though he was so busy, he was able to take time off to participate in this community service event. He talked about how being a doctor, busy as he is, is very rewarding, and he encouraged me to explore more about this profession, and other health professions. So from there, by talking to my teacher, I learned about the hospital internship, and I went for it.

Feedback

Ryan: You talked about the hospital internship, and being a scribe, and that was, in my mind, already past your decision to be a physician. Those were ways to get experience because you wanted to be a physician, but what actually brought you into medicine? And that's why I dug a little bit deeper there, and you told me that bone marrow story.

Student C: I mean, it was a combination of me being a science major, and interacting with a lot of premeds.

Ryan: So, why did you pick a science major?

Student C: Because I liked science in high school. I don't have a precise answer to why I decided to do the hospital internship. I was curious. That's the best answer.

Ryan: Why were you curious?

Student C: Because I was exposed to the talk about the premed life, and also, the leukemia, the bone marrow, and talking to the doctor. So, should I mention that?

Ryan: That's your story. Just say you've always been interested in science. You did well in science in high school, or you did well enough, or, you liked science enough in high school that you decided to be a biology major coming into college. You didn't really know what you were going to do with that, at that point, "But there was one interaction that I had with a physician at a bone marrow drive that got me interested and thinking about medicine." That's your story.

Interview 2

Student C: Besides being surrounded by premeds in my biology major, what really started the spark of my interest in medicine was when I first participated in the bone marrow drive, and I had a very detailed discussion with the attending physician there. He elaborated on certain things about finances and also the stress and the responsibilities of a doctor, and I was interested, from that discussion on. So I decided to pursue a hospital internship for two years. And doing the hospital internship, I was able to better appreciate the value of patient care. I had the opportunity to care for patients when they were down, when they were having a hard time.

I bathed the patients, fed them, cleaned them when necessary, and it was a rewarding experience just to hear their stories and how they got there and why, and what was going on with their lives. It was rewarding overall, so after that I wanted to learn more about the roles and responsibilities of a doctor, and decided to become a medical scribe for a while. And, almost embarrassingly, I wasn't able to distinguish any differences between DOs and MDs for a while. So I decided to shadow, and that allowed me to better appreciate the holistic philosophies of DOs, in particular the value of preventive medicine and also the importance of body regulation, body unity. And in particular I loved the OMT that was performed. It was very, it was very amazing to watch. And being a hands-on guy myself, doing that, it's a great tool for me to have as a doctor later on."

Feedback

Ryan: You talked about the bone marrow drive. You said that the physician talked with you about finances. Finances was the first thing that you said, so that was interesting. It made me think, "Oh, so he wants money. He's interested in money. I hope he doesn't think that you become rich when you become a physician."

So, don't mention anything about finances or money. Yes, you are paid relatively well as a physician. That doesn't mean you're rich. It doesn't mean you're wealthy.

There are a lot of medical school loans to pay back. Typically, when you look at surveys of physicians, the majority that are unhappy are typically unhappy with their pay, and their reimbursement rates. If you're going into it for money, that's a red flag, because you're typically not going to be satisfied with your pay as a physician.

Student C: I just mentioned one word, and I see that might trigger the butterfly effect and people might think I'm a greedy person. Okay, I won't mention it.

Ryan: There are many, many, many other ways to make a lot of money in this world, professions that are much easier than being a physician.

Student C: Yes. Okay, I'll keep that in mind, then, not to say anything about money, or wealth, or riches. Understood."

Ryan: Yes. "Why do you want to be a doctor?" "Because I want to drive a Ferrari." Not the right answer.

STUDENT D

Interview 1

Student D: I wish I could say that I'm like your typical student who always wanted to be a doctor their whole life or had that seminal moment, but I guess it started about five years ago. It's like a little snowball that turned into a big snowball, that led me to getting out and doing my post-baccalaureate. I was about to deploy to Afghanistan... it was about three months before I left for Afghanistan. And I was a new guy in my unit.

When you're a new guy, no one really talks to you. They were feeling me out, and I met my first good friend in the unit, who happened to be the battalion surgeon. And he was the new guy too, so as the two new guys, we just became best friends. And then when we deployed together, we ended up living together in the same tent for nine or ten months. So I ended up just literally knowing everything about the guy's job, including how he deals with the interactions between medics and nurse and PAs, and so over the course of time, I found that it would be the perfect job for me.

Ryan: I want to hear a little bit more. I'm sure lots of people have friends who are doctors but that doesn't mean they want to be doctors themselves. So there's got to be something else in there, I would think, that triggered this as well.

Student D: Well, once again, it was like a little snowball that became a huge snowball. During Afghanistan, I would literally go to his steel tent and talk to the soldiers that he helped. I would talk to the PA they worked with and the nurse they worked with as part of the team. I really probed his mind to see what it was about the job that they liked. And then we came back and redeployed to Fort Hood, and I followed him in the clinic a couple days just to see what actual garrison life was like. And I think the most important thing that I found was that as an Army doctor, you build a relationship and you help the soldier, but at no point in that relationship do you ever ask for money. There's no surprise moment where the patient gets a thousand-dollar bill and then think that I duped them. It's like, I really get to help the person with everything I do. I get to help and get no money in return, and I can't think of another job that has that kind of ability.

Feedback

Ryan: That was too short. I had to keep eliciting a little bit more. I said, "Lots of people have friends who are physicians, so there's got to be something else." I asked that follow-up question because you said there was no seminal moment, it was a little snowball, turned into a big one. "I met one of my good friends, we lived together. He was the battalion surgeon," and that was basically where you stopped. But you can add to that—you can talk about growing up, you can even talk about how your mom's a pharmacist, so there was some early healthcare exposure from the pharmacist side. You can say "My mom was a pharmacist, but I never really had the healthcare bug until I deployed and my tent mate was the battalion surgeon..."

You have a great story there for "Why medicine?" It's just a matter of formulating that good story. "Until five years ago, I thought I was going to be an Army officer for the rest of my life, doing intel stuff, but then I was exposed to my good friend, we tented together, and I shadowed him. I liked the interactions. I asked questions," and so on. You can put together a good story.

Interview 2

Student D: In 2008, I don't know if you remember this, but it was Barack Obama's speech that called people to arms to be part of the Afghanistan surge, and I joined the Army. I became an intel officer for five years. I just had this patriotism in me, I guess. So I did that for five years, and during that time period

I really found a passion for Army medicine. Then I did my post-baccalaureate work, and here I am.

Ryan: What was it about Army medicine that drew you to make that big change in your life to come back to school?

Student D: You know, it's funny, because my mom is a pharmacist, and she owned her own pharmacy with my dad. Co-located in that pharmacy there was a doctor. It was like advertising, I guess. So growing up I had a lot of access to medicine. But the truth is that five years ago was the first time I ever wanted to be a doctor. I moved into my tent in Afghanistan, I met [redacted], the battalion doctor, and we lived together in the same tent with only a six-foot plywood wall between us. You know someone extremely well, if you live like that for nine, ten months. I went to his clinic, asked the nurses, asked the medics, talked with the PAs, and just got this sense that Army medicine, and treating Army patients, soldiers, is what I really want to do.

When I got back I shadowed him a couple of times at Fort Hood, and then I moved to El Paso, Fort Bliss, and I continued my shadowing there. And it just snowballed, and I had to get out and do my post-baccalaureate work. So, that's my story in terms of becoming a doctor.

Feedback

Ryan: You talked about a speech that Obama gave, and you felt called to arms, and you joined the Army. You did a great job integrating the experience of having the battalion surgeon as your neighbor, and everything that you did to go out and seek information, seek knowledge, and build your passion for medicine. It was a great job.

Still, bring it around to why you are choosing to change careers—it's a big life decision. And you talked about your early access to medicine with your mom being a pharmacist and all that. But you really hadn't thought about it, so that was great.

CHAPTER 28

WHY NOT NURSE OR PA?

This question is similar to "Why Medicine?" We talked about some of the traps that you can fall into when answering the question "Why medicine?", and this is one of them. This is an easy question to ask students who have parents who are nurses, NPs or PAs. I often ask students with exposure to healthcare from a parent why don't they want to follow in their parent's footsteps? What is it about being a physician that makes them want to do something more?

STUDENT A

Student A: It's the idea of being in charge, having more to do, and not just being a physician's assistant. There's a lot more that I can do being a physician, rather than a nurse or a physician's assistant, so that's just one main reason for wanting to be a physician as opposed to the other healthcare professionals.

Feedback

Ryan: You talked about the nurses and the PAs and the physicians in a previous answer, which is why I then asked "Why a physician?" If you've been exposed to all of these other fields, what is drawing you towards being a physician? The answers you gave, such as being in charge—you can be in charge as a nurse. You can be in charge as a PA. Are you talking about having the final say when it comes to medical treatment? Are you talking about being in charge in a supervisory role? "Having a lot more that I can do" is what you said. In my mind, your answers didn't solidify that you really understand the differences between each of the team members—between a nurse, a PA, and a physician. So go back and try to solidify in your mind why exactly it is that being a physician is calling to you.

STUDENT B

Student B: The doctors, compared to nurses or PAs or any of those professions, to me, have a deeper level of understanding. There's a deeper knowledge of what's behind the causes. There's the ability to address unknown concerns, not just diagnose and treat, and that to me is very intriguing and one of the main reasons academic medicine is my goal.

Feedback

Ryan: It's an interesting answer, and it's one that I hear a lot from people who are thinking about changing careers from a nurse or PA to a physician. They talk about their lack of knowledge and desire to learn more. I think you did a good job addressing that without being too negative towards the other careers, which is a very common trap.

STUDENT C

Student C: That comes from the experience I had in the military. Again, it was a unique opportunity. When you're deployed you're the only one there, oftentimes. You're responsible for the care, the treatment, everything that happens to a patient.

And you have to make the tough calls, and that's something that I really thrived on. I really had a good experience, and I enjoyed doing that. When you come back to the civilian side or when you're in the country—I was in the emergency room and that's where I was assigned and I learned a lot there, in interacting with physicians, PAs, and nurses. That allowed me to discern what I wanted to do from what I didn't want to do, and that's where I discovered that osteopathic medicine was definitely the ride I wanted to take.

Feedback

Ryan: I liked what you said about all the experience that you had in the military, your being deployed and that all the responsibility is on you. You still weren't differentiating yourself too much. PAs and NPs can have a lot of responsibility. But then you finished it up by being back working in the hospital, working with nurses and PAs, and seeing all the interaction and teamwork there, so that was good. That shows me that you've experienced the range of healthcare providers out there, which is good.

CHAPTER 29

WHY DO?

This is a very specific question for interviews at DO schools. Unfortunately, there is still a stigma around DO schools and DO students. The thought that circulates among premed students is that if your grades aren't good enough to get into an MD school, then you should apply to DO schools. This thinking is bogus. Statistically, it has recently become harder to get into DO schools than MD schools. Looking at data provided by the AAMC, the acceptance rate for MD students was about 39% for 2015. That same year, the data from AACOM showed an acceptance rate of only about 31%. Yes, if you look at average GPAs and MCAT scores, they are typically lower at DO schools, but that doesn't mean it's easier to get in.

An osteopathic medical school will want to know that you want to be an osteopathic physician because of their beliefs and training styles, not just because you didn't think you could get into an MD school.

STUDENT A

Student A: I've always had a passion for health fitness, and I was an urban studies major in college, but somewhere around my junior year I decided that I didn't want to do urban studies. And I looked internally and said, what do I love to read about, what do I love to learn about, talk about? And I realized I really am interested in nutrition. I'm sorry, can you repeat your question one more time? I want to make sure I'm staying on track.

Ryan: What's your interest in osteopathic medicine?

Student A: That's right. As I explained previously, when I did that internship and I saw her practicing as an osteopath, and being able to incorporate her interest in diabetes research, while educating these women in how to live healthier, fuller lives, I saw how you can take a holistic perspective with a patient, and you're not just treating them. You're not just telling them, "You know you have to take more of this medication." You're looking at their whole life. You're looking at their environment, what they eat, how they exercise and care for themselves.

And then I did a little research, and I looked up how osteopathic manipulative medicine does that on a physical level, and I'm really interested in that. And the whole-gestalt philosophy really resonates with why I'm interested in the healthcare field and specifically why I want to treat patients. I want to address them, listen to their stories. I understand that you have to take time with patients to really tease out what it is we can do, how to provide them with the best treatment. And I feel that being an osteopath really honors my goals and values in that respect.

Feedback

Ryan: I really wasn't sure where you were going with that. And then you brought it back to the physician who you had talked about earlier. You didn't mention at first that she was an osteopath.

So when you said, "I saw her practicing as an osteopath," I thought she must have been a DO. Have you seen OMT in person? Have you seen anything like that, or have you just seen the one DO who you shadowed?

Student A: I actually had the opportunity to visit [redacted] a couple of weeks ago, and I shadowed a pediatrician there. She had the third-year students go in with the patient first and take the patient history, and they did a little bit of the manipulative medicine. Their patients were young children who were not compliant, screaming, so it was really hard for them … but they tried. So I got to see it in practice. I've read about the concept, and it has to do with structure and function, and it really makes sense to me. As an athlete, I've felt where my hips are a little out of alignment and then I go to the physical therapist. I know I'm not calling it the same name, but he'll make some adjustments so my structure is normal again. And then I'll physically feel better—my hip feels better. I feel like I've benefited from treatments similar to OMT.

Ryan: Why not talk about that?

Student A: Yes, that's a good point.

Ryan: Yes. As an athlete, you have a background of needing a lot of manipulative medicine, and you got it through your physical therapist. You can talk about how your physical therapist did some manipulations with you and that you're excited to bring that to your patients, as well as a medical background as a physician, and the other tools that you'll have at your disposal to be able to treat patients.

Knowing how it benefited you, you know it will benefit your patients. When did you first learn about osteopaths?

Student A: When I was doing my internship and shadowing Dr. [redacted], through the [redacted] Diabetes Research Institute.

Ryan: You could even talk about how you first learned about osteopathic medicine through her, and that looking back at your tennis career, you would have greatly benefited from having an osteopathic physician and add a little twist in that way.

STUDENT B

Student B: What really made me choose osteopathic medicine was the shadowing because in the hospital, I wasn't able to really distinguish between the professions. They were practically identical in what they did. Shadowing allowed me to explore more OMT in particular, and it also allowed me to discuss with the DOs about the holistic approach, the DO philosophy. What some of them said about their belief in the whole body unity, and how they believe something could have really prevented the need for medicine—I really took that to heart.

Feedback

Ryan: I like that you were honest about not really knowing the differences between MDs and DOs while you were in the hospital. It's a common thing that patients won't know the difference or what their physician actually is—an MD or a DO. Obviously, at the end of the day both MDs and DOs are physicians taking care of patients. You were able to step beyond just the title and see first-hand what the DOs do with manipulation, which is great. The discussions that you had with the DO physicians show that you've sought out the information.

STUDENT C

Student C: Well, I could really tell the difference when the physicians were treating patients. All the patients received excellent care, no matter what provider they had, allopathic or osteopathic, but I could really tell the difference just in the way the physicians treated the patient.

The osteopathic physicians would delve deeper into anything going on with the patient in terms of their physical state, and their emotional and spiritual well-being, just as a whole to try to adopt this multifaceted approach, and I really appreciated that. I thought that that was a really unique technique.

Occasionally, I'd also see them use the OMT techniques to help with earaches, or use point pressure on tenderness on any particular area of the body, and I thought that was spectacular. That's what I really like.

Feedback

Ryan: You did a good job explaining your experience and your exposures. I like that you didn't get too negative. You said, "Everybody treats everybody well, but there was just something extra that I saw with the DOs."

CHAPTER 30

WHAT IS YOUR BIGGEST WEAKNESS?

The biggest weakness question is a very popular question in interviews to see how well you know yourself and to see how much you are willing to admit about yourself. This is not the time to disguise a strength as a weakness. A very popular one is to say that you work too hard, or that you are too motivated. Below you can see some back and forth discussion on trying to get to a good answer after students give the clichéd answers first.

STUDENT A

Student A: I am a perfectionist, and I always want to do everything in my power to help my patients. Right now I'm working as a medical assistant at a surgical dermatology office, and I definitely do take my patients home with me at the end of the day. I think about what I could have said differently so they would have understood better, and how I might have communicated something a little bit more clearly. And it will bother me. I'll go to sleep thinking shoot, I wish I'd said this or didn't say that. Or I could call Mr. Jones and let him know I didn't get a chance to review his pathology with him today, I will have to wait until tomorrow. But he's probably wondering why I didn't call.

I just tend to take things away at the end of the day and not just leave them at work, even though maybe it's better for my personal well-being if they stay there.

Feedback

Ryan: So using "being a perfectionist" as your weakness would be very clichéd.

It's almost like saying "I know it's a weakness, but it's really what makes me strong, and it's how I'm able to succeed. So, I don't have any real weaknesses, I'm just awesome.'"

As you were talking more about what you do, and how your perfectionism manifests itself, I think you could easily say that you have a tendency to overanalyze situations. And while it's basically the same thing, the impact is very different.

Student A: I like that.

Ryan: You told a great story there about your patients, but see if you can talk about a situation with family or friends as well, something non-medical.

Again, you don't want to be selling yourself too much. Your job is to create as much of a conversational feeling as you can. So, when you say "I'm a perfectionist," and "I think about my patients all the time," and so on, it just concerns me that all you're trying to do is tell me stories to sell yourself as a great future physician.

It's a great story. I think it tells exactly what you're trying to say, but if you have a different situation in which you overanalyzed a particular situation with family or friends, that would be useful.

Whenever you're asked what your biggest weakness is, or your biggest strength, any challenges that you've overcome, any of those kinds of questions, it's your opportunity to say, "My biggest weakness is that I tend to overanalyze things." Give an example. Then you can say, "But I have been more aware of it lately, and here's what I do to fix the situation, and here's how I turn it into a strength. Here's how I will use it moving forward.'"

STUDENT B

Student B: What I've noticed in the past few years is that I'm very, very direct, so I come off harshly sometimes. I think that the world I was raised in, full of athletes and essentially male-dominated and even the military, just reinforced directness and honesty. And from what I've noticed, a lot of people can't take truth. I mean, you have to sway the truth around to a nicer way instead of being completely direct, even with bad news. Basically I need to soften myself a little bit in terms of interactions with people. That's what I've noticed. It's my biggest weakness right now.

Ryan: Okay. As a physician obviously you may be put in a situation where you have to deliver bad news, and if I was a patient of yours, I think I would go running for the hills if you came to me with a very direct, harsh tone or blunt direct statement. How do you take that weakness and mold it for a physician who has to build empathic relationships with his/her patients?

Student B: I'm fairly good at reading people, so in terms of military guys, and girls, I know them well. I can understand them, so I can read them. But once again, it takes practice. It takes learning. It takes constantly thinking about my actions because we all have sympathetic and parasympathetic reactions, with fast and slow reactions. So it's just a constant fight—I will always take that five seconds to think before I say anything. It's a struggle.

Feedback

Ryan: I think your answer was spot on, but I think that some of your answers come off as negative because of your biggest weakness—being very direct. You talked about being completely direct, even with bad news. That's another red flag because physicians need to be empathic, they need to have trusting relationships with patients. That's why I followed up with "How do you change that as a future physician who will need to deliver bad news often?"

I liked your answer. It's the truth. However, I might not say that you're very direct even with bad news. I think you can talk about how you know this an issue, and you're working on rectifying it by taking a pause and having that ability to respond differently.

STUDENT C

Student C: I would say the biggest weakness that I have is also useful in many circumstances. That's just my perfectionism—a high attention to detail and being really focused on everything being perfect and making things as good as I can. In a lot of ways it's helpful, but of course, it's also a hindrance. I could see specifically in medicine...If you get one-tracked, or if you get focused on one thing, or try to perfect on one thing, or work really hard, you can miss the whole big picture, which is really important in medicine. It's important to have that broad scope, and I can definitely see how that's something that I should work on specifically for medical school.

Ryan: How do you think you would work on that?

Student C: I think part of that comes with opening up. When you're in that educational experience and you're seeing patients, and keeping a focus on what you know you need to work on, so that you're paying attention to the patient as a whole, you have to take a holistic approach to what's going on with the patient and not focusing inward, or targeting one thing too specifically. Keeping an open mind.

Feedback

Ryan: This is an old, very clichéd biggest weakness: being a perfectionist.

If you haven't done this exercise, I would email friends and family who you're close to and ask them what they think your biggest weakness is, and see what they tell you.

Student C: I did that, and I got a couple of responses. Some of them I have to throw out, because I don't want to give any hint that they be an issue in medical school.

Ryan: And what are you referring to?

Student C: Indecisiveness, difficulty making decisions. When I'm considering important decisions and things like that, I often turn to friends and family. I just don't want that to come across as a negative. A lot of medicine is decision making, and it's up to you. I don't want to throw that vibe out there. In addition to the perfectionism, a lot of my friends and family referenced the "yes I can" attitude. What they meant is that anytime anyone ever asks for something, I always say yes. They think I have difficulty saying no. I weighed that as an option, and I could use that as well. Then the last answer I got was "caring too much about helping people" and I just want to avoid that altogether.

Ryan: That's another clichéd response.

Student C: That's too cliché, that's right.

Ryan: It's curious that you want to avoid the "indecisive" answer, because I think that's the best one. It all depends on how you spin it, right? What situations are you indecisive about?

Student C: "Any large decision that affects multiple people, or affects long-term things. I mean, I make fine decisions about what I'm eating and what I'm doing today, and that kind of thing.

Ryan: How long did it take you to pick out what you're wearing?

Student C: About thirty seconds.

Ryan: Okay, so I see that as a good thing. You talked about your need or want to consult with friends or family when making decisions. With healthcare now, a team approach is important in medicine. So you can spin it and talk about how you're indecisive, talk about what scenarios make you feel indecisive, describe a situation where you were indecisive, and then talk about how you think that being indecisive has allowed you to seek out others for information. You can say that their knowledge helped you make a better decision for yourself, and how in medicine, you think that would help benefit the patient when you're working with a team. That's a great way to spin indecisiveness, and it's not as clichéd as, "Oh, I'm a perfectionist."

Of course, there can be a negative connotation with indecisiveness if you don't spin it the right way. I would not say, "Oh, I take forever to make every decision, and that's just a big problem that I've always had, and I can't figure out how to fix it."

I asked you a follow-up question about your perfectionism, how you'd work on it. If they ask about a biggest weakness, or a red flag, or any problems, you must always, always offer up a spin on how you'll capitalize on it in the future, how you'll move forward. What you've learned, what you've gained. So don't make me ask you—you need to offer that answer. So, you said, "Oh, my biggest weakness is that I'm a perfectionist." Don't make me ask you how you're going to take those lessons, or what have you learned to move forward. Spin it yourself and show them that you've thought about the problem in depth, and talk about how you're going to be better as you move forward.

CHAPTER 31

WHAT IS THE BIGGEST CHALLENGE FACING HEALTHCARE?

Knowing what is going on in the world of healthcare is important before you head in for your interview. Use the major web outlets to stay informed with what is going on. Sites like KevinMD.com can also help give you some insight into the commentary outside of the normal news outlets.

STUDENT A

Student A: I would say that we need physicians who come from a variety of backgrounds and experiences and are able then to relate to their patients on a deeper level and build trust and understanding. People who understand that the physician is there to really help them, and there are no other motives in the physician being there for them, because I think especially in the more vulnerable

163

populations, there's not this trust. They've grown disillusioned with the medical system and don't feel the need to seek out care when it's necessary. So a lot of their conditions become more acute, and become harder and harder to control, but they're not seeking out medical care when they need it.

The most pressing issue is finding physicians who have this compassion and this ability to really connect with their patients, but who also really want to hear their stories and gain a deeper understanding of where the patient is coming from.

Feedback

Ryan: That is an interesting twist. You're basically saying we need more nontraditional students to become physicians. And guess who's a nontraditional student! It was a good little twist.

Student A: I'm reading God's Hotel, by Victoria Sweet. I don't know if you're familiar with that, and I wanted to go into it a bit—that was her take too, but then I didn't mention it. I don't know if you think I should or could have, or if it would have made a difference?

Ryan: You can talk about it because if you're an avid reader, talking about agreeing with an author's take is good. The person who's interviewing you might be an avid reader too, and perhaps you can have a conversation about books. It shows that you're interested enough to consume that information and read about it and do new things, so feel free. If you have that knowledge from reading a book, then share it. That's good.

STUDENT B

Student B: One of the things that I've read a lot about recently, and also heard on some of the podcasts that I've been listening to, is that there seems to be a lot of discontent in the medical field, as far as physicians go. This poses an issue for two reasons. First, there is a lack of physicians. Especially going into the future, we are going to need more physicians. And second, if those physicians are discontent, and they're telling people, "Don't come into this field because you won't be happy, or you won't be satisfied, or it's not what you expect," then, ultimately, what that leads to is a future of a growing population that needs healthcare, and a shrinking workforce to provide it. And I think that moving forward, that's one of the greatest, if not the greatest, challenges faced by the medical field.

Feedback

Ryan: That's an interesting and well-thought-out answer. It's more on the negative side as you talk about the discontent of physicians, which ultimately isn't wrong, but there are other ways of stating the same thing. You can also talk about the positive experiences you've had and why you are ignoring those physicians who are telling you to stay out of medicine. You can talk about those physicians; you can say that you don't know about the experiences that they've had, but other physicians who you've encountered, and every experience that you've had, only strengthened your desire to enter the medical field.

STUDENT C

Student C: Obviously there are a lot of challenges to healthcare. The obvious answer to me is the healthcare gap. There's an enormous gap between underprivileged populations and people that are a little more privileged, people whose health is more provided for, more taken care of. I think there are a lot of reasons that occurs. A big part of the reason is simply education. Too many underprivileged people don't realize the impact of not participating in primary care. For a lot of them, the first interaction they have with a doctor is treatment-oriented, where they're having to have surgery or they're having treatment for diabetes. Perhaps the yearly doctor's visit isn't stressed to them, and I can relate as an individual who lived in circumstances similar to that. You just don't put a priority on primary care, and when you have to drop twenty to fifty dollars for a co-pay and you're living on $200 a week, that kind of doctor's visit just takes a really low priority.

I think a lot has been done to try to address that. The Affordable Care Act is an attempt to address that and has succeeded on some levels. The impact of the cost reduction hasn't quite come to fruition, but it's a step in the right direction. I think there's a lot more that we can do to close that gap.

Feedback

Ryan: I like your comments about the healthcare gap, talking about how there are people who have healthcare, and people who don't. I like how you went into the reasoning behind this. And I agree with you—I think education is huge.

I like how you talked about the Affordable Care Act. You dipped your toes into that a little bit, and you talked about some of the negatives, how it's not reducing costs adequately.

CHAPTER 32

WHAT DO YOU THINK ABOUT THE ACA?

Similar to the above question, the Affordable Care Act (ACA), known as Obamacare, is a big topic when talking about healthcare today. You should know some pros and cons of the ACA and some of the discussions around the ACA. Using this link http://medicalschoolhq.net/acanews will open up a Google News page with a search for the Affordable Care Act to see what is being talked about. As I'm writing this there were five different articles posted within the last 24 hours. The Texture app is another great resource to stay current with what is happening in healthcare. I talked about it a lot more in the Before the Interview chapter.

STUDENT A

Student A: My friends all complained because initially we were supposed to raise the rates for primary care, but what it really did was level it, or level it to Medicaid, and then they just keep lowering the Medicaid reimbursements. So in general, this act has lowered everyone's pay, and it will continue to lower everyone's pay for some time. From a doctor's perspective, and pay-wise, I can see why they're very unhappy with it.

But as I shadow, I've seen it from the other side, where there are literally people who come in who have never had health insurance before. On one end of the spectrum, the side that's uninsured, medical bills will kill you. Once you have one huge medical bill in your debt load, you'll never get out from under. And as I get older, I understand sociology more and I understand that where you start isn't where you necessarily end, but it can help you so much to start out right at the beginning of your life. And your life shouldn't be decided because you had one accident that cost you $5,000, or one accident that cost you $10,000 in medical bills. That's where I stand. So I'm pro-Obamacare. I guess that's my final answer.

Feedback

Ryan: You said, "You know what, I see both sides." "And 'My friends all complain.'" You talked about reimbursement levels, how they're all level to Medicaid. Well, guess what? Insurance companies have paid what Medicare pays for a long time. So that's nothing new. You talked about it continuing to lower everyone's pay, and you said, "I can see why doctors are unhappy." So this is all negative, negative, negative. And then you said "I can see it from the other side," and you talked about shadowing and seeing patients who have never had insurance. So, the way to spin that again is to start on a positive note. Something like, "In my shadowing experiences, I've talked to a lot of patients (or I have seen a lot of patients) who are finally getting the medical care they need because now they have insurance that they've never had before."

And you can talk about how there are a lot of concerns, right? Not complaints. You can say "There are a lot of concerns from the physician side, from the hospital side, about certain aspects of the Affordable Care Act. But with all new things come growing pains, and I'm sure, over time, that a lot of these concerns will be worked out." By saying it this way you're highlighting the positive. You're recognizing the fact that there are some concerns and some negatives, but over time hopefully those will all work out because the positives are there.

STUDENT B

Student B: I think it's a good move. It's a move in the right direction. I think that universal healthcare is a right. Everyone should have access whether it's an emergency or they want a wellness visit. And I think the Affordable Care Act moves toward finding a balance between preventive care and trying to figure out a way to properly fund it. There are obviously a lot of opinions about it. But I think emphasizing wellness visits, and knowing that doing that and investing in that will prevent further costs, is an important move. And in general, for healthcare to focus not on when someone gets sick, but rather focus on people staying well, seeing what can we do to keep them well, is an important place to focus.

I think the cost is an issue, and what will happen with funds going for insurance companies, and how much government is involved. I think the main point is that patients should have the right to go to a doctor when they need it. There are issues with the individual mandate and all these things. But the crux of the matter is that I believe that healthcare is a right.

Ryan: Okay. So, you have a lot of positives there. What is a negative part of the Affordable Care Act?

Student B: I think the individual mandate is a little tricky. As we discussed earlier, the California case imposes on individual freedom and choice. And taxing people who don't receive healthcare? There's just a balance between the patient and the insurance companies. So, I think there's just a problem there with our value. Where we are putting the emphasis? And I think with our system, we just have so many elements going on. With the VA system, it's one thing, and then there's Medicare and Medicaid. We are trying to balance so many elements. I think some sort of integration would be better than trying to introduce even more things. There's just so much in the Affordable Care Act that it's just overwhelming for the general population to understand what it means for healthcare in America.

Feedback

Ryan: You said it's a move in the right direction, you talked about healthcare being a right for everybody. You kept talking about emphasizing wellness visits. You missed an opportunity to use the term there to easily pinpoint and talk about preventive health or preventive medicine. That's what it's all about, right?

Then I asked about the negative part of it, and again the individual mandate came up. You talked about whether it is the government's right to force someone to pay for healthcare if they don't want it. Thoughtful. You were able to talk about things, you had an opinion. It was a good answer.

STUDENT C

Student C: The Affordable Care Act represents a lot of good intentions, and I think that it's a good idea, trying to extend insurance to as many Americans as possible. There are a lot of details in there that somewhat favor the average American. Certain issues such as being denied coverage due to pre-existing conditions have been eliminated for children, at least. I think that's a really big deal. Also, insurance companies can't just spike premiums without public justification, so those are two caveats that I think make the Affordable Care Act a good idea.

There are also some downsides with the budget and perhaps insurance companies having to charge healthier patients just to take care of the sick patients. It has its pros and cons. Overall I think it's a good idea. There are a lot of kinks that need to be ironed out. And I think if our government could sit down and put their heads together, it could be around for the long haul.

Feedback

Ryan: You talked about how it represents a lot of good intentions. You talked about pre-existing conditions, for children at least. Denying coverage based on pre-existing conditions for all patients has been barred. You talked about no spike in premiums, which is good. So basically what this question told me was that you really aren't as knowledgeable as you should be with the Affordable Care Act. Most people aren't, but you need to be for the purpose of these interviews. So I would go and brush up on it. There is a good podcast episode from the Congressional Dish that you should listen to - www.congressionaldish.com/the-affordable-care-act-obamacare.

STUDENT D

Student D: There are different ways to view the Affordable Care Act, and the first way concerns how it's providing healthcare to millions of Americans—I think that's a wonderful thing. Now people are able to go to primary care physicians and have the healthcare, and have the lifestyle that they should be leading, and they can now afford that. So, that's wonderful. But with that comes increased taxes, and increased cost of healthcare for other people.

So, there are two sides to the story, and it's not a flawless system. But I definitely think that having the ability to give people the healthcare that they need at a cost that they are able to pay is wonderful.

Ryan: It's interesting. I don't remember ever seeing any ballots or any decisions being made to pay more taxes to cover the Affordable Care Act. Where does that fit in?

Student D: I read online that it has definitely increased people's insurance premiums. I know for sure that people's insurance costs might have gone up to provide insurance to those who weren't able to afford it before.

Ryan: Okay. Do you think it'll be around in four years, five years?

Student D: I think so. I think that it would be hard to take something away that has provided insurance to so many people. I think it'll be adaptable, and I think some things need to change with insurance companies too. And it's a very complicated system of paying for medical care, and I think something needs to be streamlined in order to make it simpler, or easier to use. Because even now it's still as confusing, and some care is definitely covered, but it's still not flawless so…"

Feedback

Ryan: The Affordable Care Act trips everybody up because it's a monster, and so I caught you in this area where you talking about it and I could tell you weren't a hundred percent sure about what you were saying. Part of that is to see how well you can talk about it. If you're going to go that deep, you better know some things. Make sure that you know what you're talking about and you have the facts down as best as possible. If you don't know a lot, then don't make things up. Just say you're not as well-informed as you'd like to be.

Then I asked you about the increased taxes for the ACA, and you said, "Well, I read it online…"

So just be careful. Everybody knows that we get all of our information online these days, so if you could talk about a great New York Times article or editorial on it, or reference something specific, or actually cite where you're getting it from, that would be best.

So, know Obamacare, know enough to talk a little bit about it.

I liked your answer to my follow-up question about whether it will be around in a few years and you said, "I think so." You said it's hard to take away what you've already been given, but you said, "It needs to be adaptable. It's a complicated system." Those were good answers.

CHAPTER 33

TALK ABOUT YOUR POOR GRADES

This is a similar question to red flags in your application, but when asking about red flags, they may be looking for things outside of your grades that you can talk about. You may have certain trends in your grades that you will have to explain. Maybe you had a poor semester or a bad year. You'll need to talk about what happened and why you think you've moved on from that. If you have poor grades over your entire college career, then you might not have to worry about reading this book, because you probably won't get an interview.

Medical schools use grades to try to understand your strengths as a student. If you have one bad year, but have since rebounded and have done well, you can talk about what happened during the year you did poorly. You should talk about what you learned and how you will move forward without repeating the same mistakes.

STUDENT A

Ryan: I was looking through your transcript, and I've seen some less than stellar grades in there—quite a few Ds. Can you explain what happened there?

Student A: Those are some blips in my transcript because I was coming from a small town, [redacted], to Boston, and I really went out of my comfort zone because I wanted to explore a different part of the country. I had a little trouble adjusting to the rigor of college classes. I didn't really set myself up to focus as well as I should have, and I underestimated what was required of me.

Even though I knew I wanted to be on the premed track, I admit I wasn't fully aware of just how much it would take. So I struggled a little bit sophomore year, and I had to recover pretty quickly, but I feel like I've been able to. And looking back, it was a very difficult time because I'd never had such a struggle in academics before. But now that I look back, I'm glad that it happened because it's made me a much more mature student. I was able to figure out what I needed to change about my habits, to be able to move forward despite an obstacle, and know that I could still do it. I didn't let it get to me or stop me from pursuing this.

Feedback

Ryan: When you go back and watch this part, listen to how you started off. "Those are some blips in my records because I was coming from a small town," and so on. That word "because" is very powerful.

In this situation, the word "because" is an excuse. "Because" in other situations can do a lot of other things, but in this situation it comes across as an excuse. You can say the same exact thing without that word "because" and come across a lot differently.

You can talk about the blips in your record, and then you can say, "You know what, I came from a small town in southern Alabama, and I wanted to have some diversity in seeing what else the world had to offer, so I went to school in Boston, a nice, big city on the East Coast. That adjustment—not only adjusting to college, but to city life and being around everything it had to offer—resulted in my not doing a good job managing my time and managing my priorities." You can sum up with "But you know what, I went through that rough patch, and

I figured out what I needed to do, and I think I corrected pretty well. Having gone through that, I know what the warning signs are if I fall back into those problems, so moving forward I will avoid that.'"

STUDENT B

Ryan: Looking through your transcripts, it appears that you struggled with math early on and then turned that around later on in your post-baccalaureate studies. What do you think was the cause of your early struggles in some of your classwork, and how did you turn that around later?

Student B: My first undergrad career was literally twelve years ago. School in general is not that hard—it's about being on top of your game constantly, repeating things constantly, just striving to work hard and keep learning. Quite honestly, when I was in college, I was just immature, but I've come a long way. I worked nowhere near as hard back then as I do now. I mean, I'm studying a lot more now. It's just more of a maturity issue than anything else. I was just a kid 12 years ago. I wanted to party and go to football games.

Feedback

Ryan: We talked about your poor grades as an undergrad. And here's the scenario where you have this negative word, being "immature." There are other ways to say that you were immature without saying those exact words. Right?

Student B: What is that word?

Ryan: You talked about just wanting to go to parties and go to football games. A lot of college students are immature. That doesn't mean they get bad grades. So you can talk about being distracted or not having any direction. You can say "I was directionless. I didn't really know what I wanted to do with my life."

Student B: Got it. I have meaning in my life now.

Ryan: Exactly. Now there's a switch that has turned on where you didn't have direction before. Now, you have direction. When you talk about being immature and wanting to go to parties and football games, well—I'm an adult. I like to party and go to football games too. You just don't want to give them any doubts!

CHAPTER 34

WHAT ARE YOUR THOUGHTS ON ABORTION? (AND OTHER ETHICAL AND MORAL QUESTIONS)

I have discussed the general framework around ethical questions in Section II. Go back and read that to remind yourself of how to best answer these questions.

Remember, there is no right or wrong answer. Let the interviewer understand your thought processes and always be respectful of both sides.

STUDENT A

Ryan: Any thoughts on abortion?

Student A: It's an interesting question. I'll need a moment to think about this. Let's see. As a personal opinion, I'm not really a fan of abortion, or I don't...

Well, let me rephrase. I don't think anybody's a fan of abortion, but I think there are other ways to deal with it. I feel that if a woman wants to terminate her pregnancy, in my opinion, I would just rather her deliver and give the baby up for adoption or to the foster care system.

There's a whole debate about whether the fetus is considered a human being at certain stages of the pregnancy, and that complicates things. I'm not an expert; I can't really say a fetus is a baby, a human being right from conception. I don't think I can really make that judgment call, but I feel that if a woman finds herself with an unwanted pregnancy, she should at least carry it out to the end and give the child up for adoption. There are a lot of families out there, a lot of spouses out there who are desperately seeking children. For one reason or the other they cannot have children of their own, so your unwanted baby might be a gift to somebody else. You never know. You never know what that child that you dispose of might grow up to become. Maybe somebody who changes the world in one way or another.

Feedback

Ryan: It didn't really sound like you had picked a side. You were just hedging your bets and walking down the middle. When you're asked these types of questions, we're looking for a side. We're looking for your thought process on how you came to that decision.

Student A: Okay, I have a question that I would like to ask before we move on. I don't know if I should be worried about this, but if you're asked such opinionated questions or very strong questions on topics such as euthanasia or abortion, should the interviewee be worried about whether the interviewer has opposite views? I mean, I guess that's why I stayed in the middle. Should I be worried about that or should I just take a stance, not minding whether the interviewer's perspective is different than mine?

Ryan: Here's an example. I'm pro-choice. That's my personal opinion and stance on the topic of abortion. I'm pro-choice. When I ask what your thoughts on abortion are, if you were to come right out and say, "Oh, as soon as that egg is inseminated, it's a living being, and if you ever kill that thing, then you're the devil," then yes, you should be worried about how you come across to me. But if instead you could say, "You know what, based on my religion, based on the way I was raised, based on my personal experiences, I think that every fetus should have a chance to be born and live a happy, healthy life, to parents who want the child," then you're telling me your position, you're being polite about it and giving me your reasoning, as opposed to totally shooting down the other side and saying that they're a bunch of idiots.

STUDENT B

Ryan: Tell me your thoughts on euthanasia.

Student B: It is obviously difficult for people to pick a side with euthanasia, especially since families are having to deal with so much at the time when euthanasia might be an option or something for them to consider. But, I believe that it is an individual's decision. It can be hard to think straight in those circumstances, and I think that's why it's important for people to let their families know what they would want to happen if euthanasia is an option, before anything were to happen. I think that ultimately, as difficult as it is, it's the individual's right to determine what happens. And in the case that a person cannot decide and something traumatic happens, I think it's really important to consider all the options and to consider what's best for the patient. And if there is a good chance that there will be a good life ahead, then I believe it might be good to take a chance and see what happens before going down the path of euthanasia.

Feedback

Student B: I feel like I didn't really say anything.

Ryan: Yeah, you know what, I don't think you really did either, but in the end you finally said, "You know what, ultimately it's the individual's decision." So you did answer the question, but there was a lot of fluff too.

Student B: I guess I didn't know how to elaborate.

Ryan: With these types of questions, you can try to put yourself in the patient's shoes. You could answer with something like "Euthanasia is a very hot topic; it's difficult for people to pick one side or the other. But if I were a patient dealing with a terminal illness, one that I know would kill me in six months, and before then leave me severely disabled and put lots of stress and responsibility on my family physically, mentally, and monetarily, I hope that I would have the ability to decide for myself, if and when I wanted to leave this earth." This answers the question, but in a little bit of a different way.

STUDENT C

Ryan: What do you think about abortion?

Student C: I'll come out right and say it, I am very much pro-choice, but the reason I am pro-choice is because I think that the woman is the one who brings life into the world, the woman is the one who carries the child for nine months. That's my position, even though I can see it from the other side, the father's side, where fathers say that they will be there the whole time, that they will be an awesome provider, that they will truly be the best father figure in the world. At the end of the day people change, and from what I have seen statistically and in my life, it always seems to come down on the woman in terms of care-taking, and that's across the whole lifetime of raising a child. At the end of the day I am pro-choice because the woman should have that choice.

Feedback

Ryan: In this answer, you gave me your opinion, which is good. You came right out and said "I'm pro-choice," but you didn't really give me an answer from a medical perspective, from a future physician's perspective. It's an okay answer, but if you had mentioned something about patients or having discussions with patients, it would have made the answer that much stronger. In the end, you gave your opinion, and you gave the reasoning behind it, and that's ultimately what we want.

STUDENT D

Ryan: What are your thoughts on abortion?

Student D: My personal thoughts on abortion aren't as important in the grand scheme of things as far as the needs of patients are concerned. As a physician, I personally would not perform abortions. That is not the area of medicine I would go into, it is a personal stance of mine. I value life to the utmost. As the physician of a patient, that patient may not agree, and they're allowed to not agree, and it would not influence my opinion of them. They are allowed to feel that abortion is an acceptable practice, and they are allowed to have an abortion if that's what they believe is in their best interest.

Feedback

Ryan: That was a great answer. For moral and ethical questions, there really are no right or wrong answers—the question concerns what your thought process is, whether you're able to be non-judgmental and get your point across, and you did. You could have expanded a little bit more about how even though you wouldn't perform the abortion, you would make sure that the patient received the care that they needed from a physician who would be willing to take care of them. Other than that, great answer.

STUDENT E

Ryan: California recently passed some legislation to allow euthanasia for patients in limited circumstances. Now that the whole West Coast has some form of euthanasia available, do you think it's something that every state should allow?

Student E: I want a moment to think about this. Let's see. As to whether every state should allow it, I would say, in my opinion, no. I feel maybe just for the potential of, and this might be a stretch, but maybe because of the potential for abuse by family members…They might just say the person is in a very bad state, why don't we take them out of their misery. I feel as though the situation becomes even more complicated when the patient did not provide an end-of-life directive, so making it a federal mandate or making it nationwide—I don't think it's a good idea. Maybe let California do it, and let's see how things go in California, and then we can go from there as to whether it should be a nationwide mandate. But, best case scenario, if California doesn't have any major problems with it, other states can take it on, one state at a time, and we'll see how it goes. But my personal opinion, nationwide, no it's not necessary.

Feedback

Ryan: It didn't really sound like you picked a side. You were hedging your bets and walking down the middle. When you're asked moral or ethical questions, we're looking for you to take a position. And we're looking for your thought process on how you came to that decision. I didn't know if it was because you were walking a line or if you need to read up a little bit about what euthanasia is or what laws California just passed regarding euthanasia. There are very strict guidelines on who can make these decisions and when. It's not as if your significant other could walk in and tell the doctor, "I want this person dead. Give him a pill now," and then that's what would happen. You also talked about seeing what happens in California, as if it's the first state to have euthanasia, but it certainly isn't. So it came across as though you didn't really know much about it and you were just talking without much knowledge.

STUDENT F

Ryan: There was a big news story within the last year about a woman who had brain cancer and moved to Oregon so she could end her life on her own terms. California recently passed legislation to allow some forms of euthanasia. Do you think it's something that every state should allow at this point?

Student F: In my opinion, yes, euthanasia should be legalized as an option. People worry that euthanasia affects the patients, and they fear higher suicide rates or that people would die a lot more, but from my own perspective, I feel that euthanasia hasn't been a real concern in terms of increasing patient deaths at all. Also, my personal belief is that a patient who has the mental clarity to understand his position, and who wants to die from euthanasia, should be able to. But in certain circumstances where the patient's family offers euthanasia, because they feel that it's appropriate—I feel that that's a little off limits, that the decision should be solely for the patient, not for any relatives.

Ryan: Do you think anybody should be able to go to their physician and say, "I want to die next week. Give me the pills."?

Student F: No, and from my perspective it's because euthanasia should only be done for appropriate reasons, such as the patient is in intolerable pain, or the patient feels guilty that he's such a financial burden to his family, or those sorts of extreme reasons. If a patient were to go to a doctor and just request some pills to commit suicide, flat-out suicide, that's not euthanasia, from my perspective. That's just finding a reason to commit suicide, and using a doctor as a tool for that.

Feedback

Ryan: You said, "Yes, it should be an option." There was one thing that you said that I didn't like. It really didn't make sense. You said, "but from my own perspective, I feel that euthanasia hasn't been a real concern in terms of increasing patient deaths," right?

So what you're stating is that you think, you *assume*, that euthanasia doesn't result in any sort of increase in patient deaths outside of those who really deserve it, or need it. You're entering medicine at a time when everything is driven by evidence. What does the data show? There's no more "I think" or "I feel." "I feel that this treatment is better," or "I've been doing this for ten years, and I remember it's always worked out perfectly, so this is the way I'm going to continue to do it."

So watch your verbiage on that. Your perspective on any increased/decreased patient deaths really isn't relevant in this situation. What is relevant is everything else you said about, "Yes, it should be allowed." I had to draw you out a little bit more concerning the scenarios in which you think it would be okay. So you said yes, in certain situations I think it's good—if there are patients who are suffering and in intractable pain or dying from cancer, whatever it may be.

CHAPTER 35

WHY SHOULD WE PICK YOU?

When it comes to talking about ourselves, we always seem to get tripped up. Writing about yourself in your personal statement, and talking about your strengths and why a medical school should pick you, always seem to be the most awkward moments. This is not your opportunity to brag. This is your time to confidently talk about how your personal experiences will benefit your classmates, your school, and your future patients. Why will the medical school be proud that you are an alumnus of their school? Don't talk about how motivated you are, or how determined you are—every student is motivated and determined. Talk about your personal life experiences and how they have formed you as a person.

STUDENT A

Ryan: What strengths would you bring to the class, assuming we accept you?

Student A: I think my greatest strength is that I've been a part of teams ever since I was a young child. Even growing up in a large family is like being part of a large team, and I know how to interact on an interpersonal basis. I know when it's necessary to step out and be the first to do something, but I also know when you're working with a team of really capable individuals, when it's right to step back and let others lead and just be a good follower. Be a person who supports others in their endeavors, and...Yes, I think that's a really valuable asset to any institution, but specifically at a medical school where you have a lot of really self-motivated individuals who want to do a lot of good.

Ryan: As I go back and I tell the Admissions Committee about you and why we should accept you, what one thing do you want me to relay to them on your behalf?

Student A: I think I would be honored if you would tell them that I have the potential for growth, and that I'm willing to put the work in to not only grow as an individual, but to grow as part of something larger than myself, to adapt as part of a team and to work to overcome my shortcomings.

Feedback

Ryan: So, being part of a team, obviously growing up playing soccer, you've been in team sports. Knowing when to step back, step out, step in. That is great, especially with healthcare nowadays being such a team sport as it is, so good answer.

I then followed up with, "What do you want me to relay to the Admissions Committee?" I like asking these questions back to back in mock interviews because they are basically the same questions, but they make you think a little bit differently. Sometimes we get some good answers, sometimes not. Here, we didn't get the gold. Go back and listen to this. The way it came across was basically as if you were saying "You know, I have some work to do, and I'm willing to put in the work. I'm worth the risk because I'm going to work to overcome my shortcomings." It sounded a bit odd. It came across as "Please take a chance on me...I know I have some issues, but I'll work really hard to fix them."

STUDENT B

Ryan: If we accept you as a student here, what are you going to bring to your classmates to motivate them, and help them succeed in class?

Student B: I think I can bring my energy, for sure, and I like to communicate, and I like working in groups too. I think it's a great way to succeed and bring all different aspects to the table. I enjoy working like that. So, I think I would be able to bring that community and sense of helpfulness to all of the students, because I think everyone should help each other in order to succeed, because we all have the same goal of becoming the best physicians that we can be. I think I would definitely be able to do that.

Ryan: Out of the thousands of applications that we get at this school, why should we choose you to take one of our seats?

Student B: I think both my passion and my unique background make me an interesting applicant and truly show my dedication to the field, and how I honestly want to do this as a career. Volunteering three days a week, on top of work, and also on top of secondary applications, and classes—I understand what it takes to work hard and do what I need to in order to succeed. So, I honestly believe that I would be a great asset to your school as a student and a dedicated premedical student.

Feedback

Ryan: The initial question about what you would bring to your classmates— you answered this by talking about energy, communication, and working in groups. In this question, you didn't highlight your unique background, but in the follow-up question you did.

What you bring to the class is *you*. You are a nontraditional applicant. You're an engineer. You need to work in groups as an engineer. You need to do all this other cool stuff. What have you done that probably ninety-nine percent of the other students in that class have not done? You'll be very unlikely to find another engineer in your class who is changing careers this way.

So, highlight you. When you're asked what will you bring, why we should pick you, talk about your nontraditional path. You've experienced a lot more, such as the challenges you've experienced because you were out in the workforce and not a traditional student.

You said something about working hard, and I made a note that "everybody works hard for this." You were angling for the idea that you possibly worked harder than anybody else. You're more dedicated than anybody else because you're working, you're volunteering, you're applying…

I would venture a guess that a lot of students are working, applying, and volunteering. So be careful about going down that route of "Look how hard I worked. I submitted my applications on time, and I submitted my secondary applications, and look at me." There 60,000-plus other students who are applying who also had to submit their applications and may be going to school instead of working full-time, whatever it may be.

So again, what's unique about you? That's what you need to focus on. The "I worked harder" line is a "better" statement—I'm "better" than that other student. We want to focus on how you are different, not better. Different is better than better!

STUDENT C

Ryan: If you're accepted here next year, what characteristics, what traits, what strengths would you bring to your classmates?

Student C: The thing that I'm proudest of is my cultural heritage. Being in Vietnam for twelve years before coming to the States, I saw healthcare in Vietnam for a while, and how horrendous the healthcare in Vietnam is in comparison to the States—patients sharing two beds sometimes, which is absurd. And by going to my class and maybe talking about it and expressing what I've experienced, I might be able to improve the diversity of the student body by allowing the other students to see what's going on in other places in the world. I also hope to bring my passion for medicine, my ability to work hard and drive others to succeed. And in particular, because of my past experiences with various clubs, I like to work with other people. At your school, you utilize inter-professional education. With my background working with other people, I feel that this will hopefully enhance the team-based environment of healthcare at your school.

Feedback

Ryan: I like your cultural heritage discussion.

You finished by talking about passion for medicine, working hard, driving others to succeed. That's very generic, and you're telling me how awesome you are instead of showing me.

Give me a little story about how you've worked as part of a team before and have driven others to succeed. Do you have a scenario or a story that you can tell?

Student C: Yes, I actually do have a scenario about that. I don't know why I didn't use it.

Ryan: That's why we practice! So when you're asked that kind of question, that's how to answer it. Give me a good story that shows what kind of leader you are, shows what kind of motivator you are, shows me how driven you are.

STUDENT D

The next two answers are from the same student over two different interviews.

Interview 1

Ryan: If you're accepted here, what will you bring to your classmates to help them achieve the best success that they can?

Student D: I think that the one thing I will bring is perspective. Being an older applicant and actually being an alumnus from this school (which is like forty percent of the class), having traveled all over Asia and Europe, to many different towns I never would've thought of while in the Army, and having tried to learn a couple of languages, I think I can give them good advice in terms of finances and just life decisions and just bring a completely new perspective to the medical school class.

Ryan: As we finish up here, I need to go back and explain to the other Admissions Committee members why we should give you a seat for our class next year. What do you want me to tell them on your behalf?

Student D: I love [this school]. This is my number one choice. I think that I fit perfectly with the mission. I want to be in primary care. I want to live in Florida in the future, not immediately of course. And I think that I bring a unique perspective to the class, and fifteen to twenty years from now, I'll be a good alum. You'll see me around consistently and persistently, and I could see myself being an associate professor somewhere and having [this school's] students following me in the future at some of the satellite campuses.

Feedback

Ryan: You spoke about the most significant thing that you'll bring—a different perspective. You're a nontraditional student; you were in the Army. You've had life experiences that a lot of students probably won't have, so you can highlight those, which you did a little bit there, so that's good. Then I asked you what you want me to tell the Admissions Committee, and you talked about how you love [this school], and how you fit perfectly with their mission. But that made me wonder if you really know what the mission is, because you didn't really tell me anything about it, except for that you "fit perfectly" with it.

You talked about bringing your unique perspective, which you do, and then you gave that fifteen- to twenty-year answer about being a good alumnus. I want you to be a good alumnus from the day you graduate!

Interview 2

Ryan: If you are accepted here, what will you bring to your classmates to help support them, to help motivate them, and to help them succeed on their journey?

Student D: I think that what I bring to the table, in terms of the class, is team spirit, and a different perspective: I have seen life and death situations, and I have traveled all over the world, so I would bring this new perspective and insight to all of my classmates. And, at the same time, I think that I am a good leader, and [this school] seems to want that. In fact, they put us in a thirty student small group for our first two years. And, I think I can truly lead that group. Because for my whole life, whether I was on a hockey team, lacrosse team, Army infantry team, or intelligence team, I've always been an integral part, and I've always built the family where I've been. So, I think that may be the most important aspect I bring.

Ryan: Is there anything else that you would want me to tell the Admissions Committee as I go back with them and review your application?

Student D: I think I fit [this school's] mold perfectly. I want to do primary care. I want to serve the underserved, and I want to live in a smaller town in Florida. I think that is where my future will be. And, at the end of the day, this is my number one choice. I mean if you told me tomorrow I could drop all of my other applications, send in my down payment, hell, I've talked to my Army recruiter, I would put my next year's tuition down tomorrow—I would. That's how serious I am.

Feedback

Ryan: Great answer here, talking about team spirit from your perspective seeing life and death scenarios. You talked about being a good leader, and I started to take notes waiting for you to tell me who you have led, or what you have led. Obviously, with your Army experience, you have had experiences leading people, and you went into that by talking about lacrosse and hockey, and then you started talking about the military. You need to lead with your military experience—it's great experience which very few applicants are going to have.

Then, don't tell me that you are a good leader, show me. Be descriptive. You can say, "I've led a battalion of ten people," or whatever it may be.

I then followed up with the question about what you want me to tell the Admissions Committee. You talked about fitting the school's mold perfectly. You're interested in primary care and the underserved. You let them know that they are your number one choice, which is fine.

Student D: Could the answer be better? Because I know that they'll ask that.

Ryan: With the previous question about what you will bring to your classmates, you can weave that one into this by talking about how you fit their mold, how they are your number one choice, and you feel that you would be an asset to your classmates, because of your perspective and the experiences that you've had outside of school. Remember that the Admissions Committee is trying to build a small community, and they want to make sure that everyone is going to fit together, and that everyone has a specific role. So your role is going to be the Army dad who is going to get everybody in line and do PT at 4:30 in the morning!

STUDENT E

The next two answers are from the same student over two different interviews.

Interview 1

Ryan: What do you want me to tell the Admissions Committee? After I leave here I have to go talk to them and try to convince them that you deserve a seat at this school. What do you want me to convey to them on your behalf?

Student E: I would say I'm dedicated to making this dream happen. This has been a childhood dream of mine, and though I've encountered many obstacles along the way, I've stuck to it and it's been rewarding to see it through, to see success. It's an honor to be invited so early for an interview, and that is really encouraging to me. To be able to succeed as a student first and foremost, and to be able to do my best to become a committed physician in this community, in Alabama, or wherever else I may practice—that's what's important.

Feedback

Ryan: At the beginning it was mostly about you, how it was your childhood dream, how you've overcome the obstacles, and how you're dedicated to making this happen. That's the stereotypical answer that everybody gives. It doesn't say anything distinctive about you.

But then you said something new, when you said, "I'll be a committed physician to the community, to Alabama," which is good. What are you going to bring to your classmates? How are you going to strengthen them? What experiences have you had in life to help you strengthen them? That's the kind of material that you should add to this answer as well.

Remember, they're trying to build a little mini community of students. They want to make sure everybody sings Kumbaya together. And if you're somebody who has had experiences which can add to their community, that makes you a better candidate.

Interview 2

Ryan: As I go back and tell your story to the rest of the Admissions Committee, what do you want me to tell them on your behalf?

Student E: I would appreciate if you would tell them how my diverse educational background and personal background have formed me into the applicant I am today. I've been able to go to a liberal arts college as well as a small town, a local university, as well as [redacted], which is a huge public university, and I've been able to study child development and do my premed requirements and form a holistic perspective of a patient. Treating the patient on a person-to-person basis, and not categorizing a child who might have autism as an autistic child, but a child with autism—that's something that I really took away from my studies. I know that is something that I will really carry with me; it really formed the way that I approached my studies.

Feedback

Ryan: You talked about your diverse background. I liked how you started with, "I'd appreciate it if you would..." That's very polite. I loved your finishing statement with the autistic child versus child with autism.

STUDENT F

The next two answers are from the same student over two different interviews.

Interview 1

Ryan: As we finish up here, I need to go and discuss your application with the Admissions Committee. I need to tell them why I think you should have a seat here at our school next year. What do you want me to tell them on your behalf?

Student F: I want you to tell them about my compassion for people and how my clinical experience reflects how I could make an excellent physician one day. I want you to tell them that I'm creative in terms of painting and my culinary adventures. And I want you to tell them that I love to learn and I'm inquisitive. I love working with others as a team, and I think those are all very valuable attributes to have as a future leader in healthcare. I want you to tell them that I am a hard-worker, and I am focused and dedicated to doing what it takes to become a physician, and to discovering how I can best serve this community.

Feedback

Ryan: So this was just a big list of telling me things…that you have compassion, that you're going to make an excellent physician, that you're creative, you love to learn, you're inquisitive, you love working with others, you're a hard worker, that all of these are valuable in healthcare today. I was feverishly typing all of these down. So lots of *telling* right? *Telling, telling, telling, telling.* You're a nontraditional student. What you should be telling the Admissions Committee is what you bring to the diversity of the class. How that diversity may help your classmates. How it will help the university and how it will help your patients. Those are the things that you should be showing me through stories.

You talked about your leadership abilities. What about them? Talk about tennis and some stories from tennis in which you needed to use your leadership skills to thrive and survive. More storytelling and less just telling me all of the key qualities that you have.

I'm sitting down with you right now, and next I'm sitting down with Tom, and then I'm sitting down with Natalie. And they all say that they're hardworking. And they all say that they're passionate. And they all say that they love learning. But when you're able to tell me a story about your passion and your love for learning and your leadership ability, that stays with me instead of this list of words.

Student F: I'm kind of trying to think of what story I could tell that would integrate a lot of those qualities.

Ryan: Well, I say story but it doesn't really have to be a story. You can just say "Because I am a nontraditional student, I've had a lot of experiences outside of the classroom doing x, y, and z which I think could help my classmates next year. I think my time as a competitive tennis player and my time as the captain of a tennis team helped me hone some leadership skills which could help my classmates."

Student F: I see.

Ryan: "I think my Renaissance background allows me to connect with a wide range of patients and people" and so on.

Interview 2

Ryan: Okay. If you're accepted to next year's class, what will you bring to your classmates and to the university? What will you do to better everyone here?

Student F: When I was a freshman in college I tore my rotator cuff, and I went to the doctor. He told me I wouldn't be able to play competitive tennis again. Well I shed a couple of tears and then said, "You know what? That can't be." And I worked so hard for three months straight just doing intensive physical therapy. When I finally got back on the court at the beginning of fall semester in my sophomore year, I was staying late every day after practice. I was going to the gym doing extra workouts, I was training with the cross country team and running to build my endurance. I even made friends on the men's team and played matches with them on the weekends. And I just did everything in my power to improve so my quality of game wouldn't suffer when I got back to playing.

But I wanted to even improve upon that, and I did. I persevered through this physical and mentally challenging time to be successful. I feel like that perseverance and that determination are a huge part of why I am successful in almost anything I do. It's not that I'm a natural, it's not that I'm...I mean obviously maybe there's some talent, but I think it's really just hard work, dedication, and perseverance. And those are some of the qualities that I think I'll bring to the class among others. But I think that really stands out in my mind.

Feedback

Ryan: You had a good story here from when you were a freshman in college, but ultimately the question I had was how are you going to use your strengths to help your classmates? What do you bring to make them better? You did show me with a story, though, as opposed to just telling me. That was much more memorable for me. But in the end I don't' think you answered the question.

STUDENT G

The next two answers are from the same student over two different interviews.

Interview 1

Ryan: As we finish up here, I need to go back and tell your story to rest of the Admissions Committee members and let them know why you should have a seat here at this school. What do you want me to tell them on your behalf?

Student G: I would say that there's always a gamble on the Admissions Committee side of things, when you're looking at an applicant and deciding whether or not you should take them. One of those biggest gambles is whether this person is committed. Do they have what it takes to go through these next four years at our University, and the commitment to know that that's what they want to do, and that they're going to want to pursue it afterwards, and help this country during this shortage of physicians that we have? And I think that's my biggest strong suit here—my commitment to medicine, and the fact that I have such significant experience, from multiple sides, including direct patient care and responsibility. I think that's an important advantage, and I think it's a distinction that sets me apart from all the other applicants.

Feedback

Ryan: I loved your answer to this question. I don't necessarily like how it started. There's this weird thing where you, as the applicant, are telling me as the Admissions Committee member what my job is like. You said something like, "It's always a gamble when you are looking at an applicant" and I'm thinking, "Yes. Yes, I know. That's my job, that's why I'm interviewing you right now." You didn't need that first line in there. But everything else that you said was great—about your commitment to medicine, with all your experience with direct patient care. And you ended it by saying, "That's a distinction that sets me apart." I thought that was all strong, but again, you didn't need the beginning there.

Interview 2

Ryan: What would you bring to the class of 2016, assuming that you're accepted?

Student G: I think I'd bring a breadth of knowledge, experience, and diversity that not many other students can bring to the class. I think it's important to have background experience with different races, religions, ethnicities, and sexual orientations. If you do, you can help your classmates while you are learning about medicine and learning about how to be a good physician. You never know what kind of patient you're going to see. If you're a physician in the Middle East, 90% of your patients are going to be Middle Eastern. In the United States, you can see 10 patients, and they can be from 10 different backgrounds. I think it's important to have an understanding of different backgrounds. I also think that my background, especially my sexual orientation and my religious background, can help increase diversity here.

Ryan: Kind of along the same lines, I need to sell you to the Admissions Committee. What one thing do you want me to tell them that I can't find in your application?

Student G: I have had a lot of experience in the medical field both with one-on-one patient encounters, being a provider, as well as shadowing physicians, and I know wholeheartedly that I want to be a physician, and there's no doubt in my mind that I can be a great physician. I also know that I will spend my career working as a physician, and I think that's very important, and that sets me apart from other students who may not necessarily know 100% that this is what they want to do.

Feedback

Ryan: So you talked about your breadth of knowledge, experience and diversity. You told me that stuff, but *show* me instead. Show me more. Like breadth of knowledge of what? Your experience of what? Doing what? Your diversity of what? You can say, "I bring a breadth of knowledge, having been a medic in the Army, having been x, y, z, having traveled the world, and having treated all sorts of populations in the Army." Now, that leaves me with vivid examples of what you'll bring to the class.

I followed up with what you want me to tell the Admissions Committee. It's a hard question because it's a similar question to what will you bring to the class. But it's different enough, and your answer doesn't set you apart. That's my goal here—give me something that sets you apart. Knowing that you want to be a physician is great, but I would hope that 100% of the people that I interview want to be a physician. We need to come up with a better answer for this question. Even if you almost repeat what you just said, "Well, as I had just mentioned, my breadth of knowledge (and blah, blah, blah) all set me apart from my peers. These unique qualities are what also allow me to help them, but I think they set me apart and make me a great candidate."

CLOSING

I've given you the knowledge to do your best on interview day. It's up to you now to take this information and put it to use. Starting now you should be figuring out who you are—you need to know what your strengths and weaknesses are. You need to start practicing speaking without using filler words like 'ums' and 'ahs.' You need to find an advisor or mentor who knows this process and sit down with them to go through a mock interview. Take some of the questions from Section II, and sit down and record yourself answering them.

As you get closer to your interview day, reread your application, know it inside and out. Make sure that you know your travel plans and that everything is ready to go. Double check that your suit fits and that your dress shoes are comfortable and fit well. Make sure that you have enough available credit on your credit cards or enough money in the bank to pay for your expenses while you are traveling.

Know why you are at the particular medical school where you are interviewing. Why do you want to go there? Know what questions you are going to ask the interviewer. Have questions ready for the medical students.

Doing each of these things will ensure that you are as prepared as you can be for your interview. Remember that your interview is the last big challenge on your journey to medical school. Why put all of your hard work in jeopardy by not being as prepared as possible?

On your interview day, take a couple of minutes to read this ending for some last minute motivation. Take a picture of the next page with your phone so you have it with you whenever you need it.

Today is YOUR day.

Today you are going to impress.

You have worked so hard to get to this point.

You deserve to be here.

You have prepared well.

You are ready.

Take a breath.

Stand tall.

Be confident.

Smile.

Relax.

Have fun.

You got this!

ABOUT THE AUTHOR

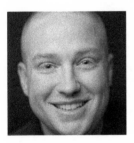

Dr. Ryan Gray is a former United States Air Force Flight Surgeon who found a passion for helping premed students on their journey to medical school. Best known for his podcasts, which have been downloaded over 1,000,000 times, Dr. Gray has interviewed numerous admissions committee members and deans of admissions for medical schools. Through The Premed Years podcast and the Medical School Headquarters sites, Dr. Gray has helped thousands of students gain the confidence they require to successfully navigate the premed path. Dr. Gray lives outside of Boulder, CO with his wife Allison, who is a Neurologist, and their daughter Hannah.

RESOURCES

MEDICAL SCHOOL HEADQUARTERS

The Medical School Headquarters consists of multiple websites and podcasts.

Websites

Medical School Headquarters: For the best information to help premeds on the path to medical school - http://medicalschoolhq.net/book/

OldPreMeds: For the nontraditional premed student on the path to medical school - http://www.oldpremeds.org/book

Podcasts

The Premed Years - http://medicalschoolhq.net/subscribe

OldPreMeds Podcast - http://www.oldpremeds.org/subscribe

POSTS ABOUT THE THE MEDICAL SCHOOL INTERVIEW

Medical School Interviews – 10 Commonly Asked Questions (http://medicalschoolhq.net/medical-school-interviews-10-commonly-asked-questions/)

Ten Medical School Interview Tips – Go in Ahead of the Competition (http://medicalschoolhq.net/ten-medical-school-interview-tips/)

EPISODES ABOUT THE MEDICAL SCHOOL INTERVIEW

The Premed Years

Session 19: Interview with a Medical School Interview and Admissions Expert (http://medicalschoolhq.net/19)

Session 91: Preparing for the Medical School Interview (http://medicalschoolhq.net/91)

Session 146: Common Medical School Interview Mistakes and How to Fix Them (http://medicalschoolhq.net/146)

Session 164: Medical Ethics Questions You Can Expect In Your Interview (http://medicalschoolhq.net/164)

Session 152: The MMI – Everything You Need to Know About the Interview (http://medicalschoolhq.net/152)

Session 191: Medical School Interview Q&A (http://medicalschoolhq.net/191)

Session 192: The Medical School Interview - How to Talk About You (http://medicalschoolhq.net/192)

OldPreMeds Podcast

Session 16: When Should I Expect an Interview or to Be Told I'm Rejected? (http://opmpodcast.com/16)

Session 30: A Statement Made About How Important Interviews Are (http://opmpodcast.com/30)

Session 31: Committee Feedback on a Bombed Med School Interview (http://opmpodcast.com/31)

Session 32: How do I Prepare for the Medical School Interview? (http://opmpodcast.com/32)

AAMC AND AACOMAS RESOURCES

Medical School Admissions Requirements – http://medicalschoolhq.net/msar

College Information Book – http://medicalschoolhq.net/cib

MSHQ INTERVIEW PLATFORM

http://medicalschoolhq.net/interview

Setting up the video camera, using flashcards for questions and recording yourself can be a pain and doesn't do the best job at simulating an interview. Our new platform lets you log into our site and use your webcam to answer premade interview sets or interviews that you build yourself with hundreds of potential questions. Check out the link above for more details on how you can get started now.

INTERVIEW PREP COURSE

http://medicalschoolhq.net/interviewcourse

Want more in-depth information, but don't need the personal, one-on-one guidance from Dr. Gray? Check out the link above to see how our video series can help you even more.

ONE-ON-ONE INTERVIEW PREP

http://medicalschoolhq.net/mock-interview-prep

Want to work directly with Dr. Gray to help prepare for your interviews? Check out the many different services available by visiting the link above.

REFERENCES

1. Admissions Office, Albert Einstein College of Medicine of Yeshiva University, 2015-2016 Applicant Guide Einstein M.D. Program, https://www.einstein.yu.edu/uploadedFiles/education/md-program/admissions/2015-2016-Applicant-Guide.pdf (accessed July 11, 2016).

2. AAMC Medical School Admissions Requirements, https://students-residents.aamc.org (accessed July 11, 2016)

3. AACOM Osteopathic Medical College Information Book, http://www.aacom.org/news-and-events/publications/cib (accessed July 11, 2016)

4. AAMC Table A-1: U.S. Medical School Applications and Matriculants by School, State of Legal Residence, and Sex, 2015-2016, https://www.aamc.org/download/321442/data/factstablea1.pdf (accessed July 11, 2016)

5. AACOM Four Year Applicant Profile Entering Classes 2012 – 2015, http://www.aacom.org/docs/default-source/data-and-trends/2012-15-app-report.pdf?sfvrsn=10 (accessed July 11, 2016)

6. University of Washington, Advocating for Equal Access, https://www.washington.edu/boundless/advocating-for-equal-access/ (accessed July 11, 2016)

7. AAMC Core Competencies for Entering Medical Students, https://www.aamc.org/initiatives/admissionsinitiative/competencies/ (accessed July 11, 2016)

8. AAMC Holistic Review, https://www.aamc.org/initiatives/holisticreview/ (accessed July 11, 2016)

9. Texture, http://www.medicalschoolhq.net/texture (accessed July 11, 2016)

10. TED Your body language shapes who you are, https://www.ted.com/talks/amy_cuddy_your_body_language_shapes_who_you_are (accessed July 11, 2016)

11. How Many Seconds to a First Impression?, http://www.psychologicalscience.org/index.php/publications/observer/2006/july-06/how-many-seconds-to-a-first-impression.html (accessed July 11, 2016)

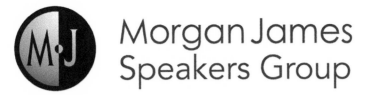

Morgan James
Speakers Group

www.TheMorganJamesSpeakersGroup.com

We connect Morgan James published
authors with live and online events
and audiences whom will benefit
from their expertise.

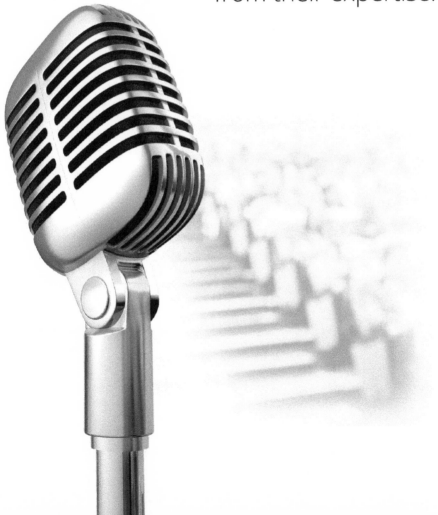

Morgan James makes all of our titles available
through the Library for All Charity Organization.

www.LibraryForAll.org

CPSIA information can be obtained
at www.ICGtesting.com
Printed in the USA
JSHW041448310820
7566JS00001B/41

9 781683 502159